GW01032998

The Aging Man's
Survival Guide

From Fitness & Finance to Sex & Sickness

JOAKIM LLOYD RABOFF

The Aging Man's Survival Guide
Concieved and written by Joakim Lloyd Raboff
www.raboff.com
© 2024 Joakim Lloyd Raboff

Graphic Design: David Pahmp
www.mediakonsortiet.se

ISBN: 978-91-989681-0-1

ABOUT THE AUTHOR

Joakim Lloyd Raboff was born in Santa Monica, California, in 1963. He has been a freelance writer, filmmaker, photographer, and visual arts consultant for the majority of his professional life.

As a teenager in the late 1970s, Joakim relocated to his mother's native Sweden, but he has also lived and worked in Spain, Thailand, Portugal, as well as in his native USA.

Joakim has produced and contributed to dozens of books, and his portfolio showcases a variety of creative projects commissioned by Swedish and international brands and organizations, including the United Nations in New York.

Each project is a reflection of Joakim's deep engagement with the subjects he focuses on.

His own personal experiences with aging played a pivotal role in the creation of this book.

DISCLAIMER

The content of this book, "The Aging Man's Survival Guide," is based on the author's 60 years of life experience, online research, and personal reflections. While efforts have been made to ensure the accuracy and completeness of the book's information, the author and publisher assume no responsibility for errors, omissions, or contrary interpretations of any of the book's subject matter.

This book also contains several references to personal anecdotes and opinions, which are subjective in nature. The inclusion of such content is meant to share personal insights and is not intended as definitive guidance for all readers.

The book provides advice on a variety of topics, including but not limited to retirement planning, maintaining relevance, increasing emotional well-being, fitness, general health, sexual health, and psychological aspects of aging. It is important to consult with appropriate professionals (financial advisors, mental health professionals, etc.) when making important decisions within these topics.

Readers are encouraged to consult with their healthcare providers before making any changes to their health routines and strategies or if they have any concerns regarding their health. The use of any information provided in this book is solely at the reader's own risk.

Lastly, the book discusses various health-related topics that might be sensitive for some readers. It is advised that individuals who are uncomfortable with such topics or who have pre-existing health anxieties or concerns proceed with caution or seek professional support.

By reading this book, you acknowledge that you understand and agree to this disclaimer.

CONTENTS

The Aging Man's Survival Guide

WHY DIDN'T I GET THE MEMO?

Dear Reader, let me start by thanking you for investing your time and money in buying, reading, or gifting this book. In it I will share some of my personal journey and reflections of turning 60 as well as a plethora of research-based knowledge and advice about male aging.

I feel confident that my exploration into what it means to be a man in his early 60s will not only resonate with many of my brethren, but also interest women by offering them insight and hopefully a deeper understanding of how aging affects us similarly to how menopause affects them. Lofty as it may sound, from the get-go, my main motivation for writing this book has been to initiate an open-minded discussion about the natural but often ignored or circumvented topic of male aging. I began writing it about a month after turning 60, in the late summer of 2023, while at a hotel on the Greek island of Rhodes. My hope was to have written the book's outline before checking out a week later, which I miraculously accomplished. When not working on the outline, I spent plenty of time pondering life and considering whether writing about my personal aging experiences would be relevant and possibly even helpful to men my age. Clearly, I must have come to the conclusion that it would.

One morning, a British fellow named Johnny, strolled into the hotel's mostly empty lounge where I had set up my makeshift writer's den. I was the only other guest there at the time, and Johnny, roughly my age, eventually came up and asked what I was working on. I read him a few lines of my outline, and he smiled approvingly before saying,

– NOW, THAT'S A BOOK I NEED TO READ.

The book's genesis, its seed, had actually begun germinating some ten years before that week in Greece. It was just as I was about to turn 50 (an angst-filled occasion in itself) while living in my native Los Angeles, when I began feeling strangely tired and sleep-deprived even after I'd slept for seven or eight hours. My previously reliable capacity to work at least 60-70 hours a week – without much rest – was no longer as easy to muster as it had once been.

BUT THERE WERE OTHER SIGNS AS WELL.

Throughout a couple of months during the fall of 2013, the fatigue I had initially experienced was also accompanied by a strange and very unfamiliar mental and physical rigidity.

This feeling came and went during the first couple of hours of most days and though I never felt sick or had any typical flu-like symptoms, it was still as if I was stuck in quicksand. I could move and think, but my usual energy wasn't there. Feeling this way was disconcerting and even somewhat worrisome. When I would normally spring out of bed just before sunrise, get into my wetsuit and jog down to the beach with a longboard under my arm, looking forward to an hour of surfing north of the Santa Monica Pier, instead I would feel so fatigued, that I wouldn't get up until 9:00 or 9:30 am. Way too late for surfing at my favorite spot.

Finally, since I'd always been able to sleep a full night without interruption, it was when I began having to get up to pee in the middle of the night that I became a little suspicious that I might actually be heading into a new phase of life.

I was still going to be in a stage of denial for several years to come and look upon these symptoms more as temporary rather than proof that a life-changing shift was afoot. In retrospect, I was clearly experiencing the first stages of male menopause, or "andropause" as it's called medically.

As I turned 55, despite mostly feeling like I was still 35, at least mentally, there was no longer any question that I was, in fact, getting noticeably older. While the rigidity had subsided a bit, or, I had at least adapted to it, there were now several irrefutable signs in my face and body that I was in fact transitioning into an older man. *I can still remember having a minor panic attack from thinking how I in 10 years time would actually be, at least societally, considered a senior citizen.*

As painful and difficult as this admission was, coupled with thoughts of how to avoid aging quicker than necessary, got me thinking about how it was probably time to start taking better care of myself. That I should no longer neglect my body's need for sufficient sleep, how getting regular exercise would probably improve my ability to cope with aging, and that I should be eating healthier and indulging less in destructive habits, including working too much.

Once I was prepared to face that I was in fact getting older, however foreign that can still be to comprehend, an urge arose to confide my experiences with a few of my oldest male friends, all the same age as me.

But without exception, every attempt I made to bring this topic up, the response I received in return indicated one of three alternatives: There was a lack of interest.

They couldn't relate at all to what I was talking about or going through.

Just like I had been, my buddies were deep in "denial land".

After researching male aging online, I found that even though 100% of all men go through some kind of andropause – male menopause – , affecting them physically, mentally, emotionally, sexually and existentially, most men are not at all interested in revealing or talking about what they're going through in this stage of their lives.

I have never participated in any of the class reunions to which I have been invited. Why? Well, primarily because meeting people I haven't seen in 40 or even 50 years is only mildly interesting to me.

Since we no longer look anything like we did as kids, what little we still have in common just isn't enough for me to make the effort it means to partake. Whatever curiosity I might have about someone from my childhood years can usually be satisfied with a look online.

Meeting people who were once as young as I was but who have now aged almost beyond recognition, myself included, seems like a depression-inducing activity that will likely only serve as more irrefutable evidence of my own physical demise.

Conversely, four of my oldest friends and I communicate almost daily (chat) and we get together for a meal or a round of drinks about once a year or so. And while we don't talk at all about how aging affects us on a physiological or psychological level, we have recently begun discussing retirement plans from a practical and financial perspective. So there's hope.

TABOO

I'm not entirely comfortable labeling male menopause a taboo topic, but that's essentially what it is. And as hard as it was to accept on a personal level, I've subsequently come to understand that we men in general, regardless of culture, ethnicity, or religion, prefer not sharing our aging experiences with each other – or with anybody.

This has been one of several incentives for me to write this book.
Depression Light

At some point during those first couple of years while I was realizing and admitting what I was going through, I began to feel a bit depressed. It wasn't debilitating, more as if I was lugging around a hefty mental backpack filled with thoughts of existential worry. Worry about how worse things might get as I continued to age. Worry about getting really sick and yes, I was worrying about dying and how that final scenario would play out.

It was also a feeling of loss as well as a fear of changing into someone unfamiliar. What could I count on keeping and what would eventually fade away from the buffet of my life? How could I possibly adjust to slowing down and not being able to get so much done?

How soon would my career be over if I could no longer keep up with younger competitors in my field of Visual Artistry? How soon would I be referred to as an old man and have younger folks offer me their seat on a bus or train? When my sex drive starts plummeting, how will it affect me?

All this extra weight felt heavy, and thinking about it would often cast a long dark shadow over my daily life. Especially when things weren't going my way or when I reached emotional hurdles that seemed higher and harder to overcome than before.

Thankfully, I never felt mentally paralyzed. Sluggish, yes. But not so much that I had to take any medication or undergo psychoanalysis. I did eventually see an anxious psychologist (are there really any other kind?) who herself was in the midst of menopause and on top of that unfortunately had very little aptitude for her profession. But it was still cathartic to open up about my feelings from within the process I was going through. For some reason, it was especially easy to do so to a woman about my age (insert Freud's Oidipus complex theory here, if you wish).

A question that still refused to leave me was why some thoughtful, older friend or relative of mine hadn't told me about how weird it was going to be to get older and how the changes in my physical appearance, the gravitational pull if you will, would slowly but surely transform me to such a degree that there would eventually only be a vague resemblance of what I looked like in younger years?

Of course, like everyone else, I've always known that aging was a natural part of life and that if you're lucky and live long enough, you'll eventually grow old. That's just logical. But even though I've had parents, grandparents, and older relatives, some even in their late 90s (and even one family friend in his early 100s), it's my own aging process that has proven to be both the most apparent and the toughest to accept.

Even today, halfway into my 61st year, with a few exceptions, each visit to the mirror is an all-too-vivid reminder of how vintage I've become. The silver lining is that as my eyesight dwindles with age, my ability (and possibly willingness) to see aging signs has also weakened.

While this slow but steady deterioration process doesn't ever really stop (until, well, you know when…), it definitely does slow down, making aging feel easier to accept and live with. And as you read on, you will find a plethora of thoughts and creative ideas for how to slow it down even more.

The overriding objective of this book is to help my fellow man recognize, understand, and hopefully deal with some of the many things that happen with us as we men age. By extension, after reading it, I hope that female companions, friends, and family members will also gain insight into the complexities of male menopause.

While not intended to be an all-encompassing guide, I certainly hope you see this book as a collection of valuable insights sprinkled with stats and facts of things to expect but not to worry too much about.

And though not everybody will recognize themselves in all of my personal experiences or the facts collected from various sources, there will definitely be plenty of valuable information for you to identify with and cherry-pick from. If not, well, then at least writing this book has helped me deal, cathartically, with my own aging process.

This book is dedicated to my friends and family who have encouraged me to write this book and have patiently awaited its completion. Special thanks to Charlotte Raboff, Elle Raboff, and David Pahmp for all their insightful help and creative input.

Joakim Lloyd Raboff, 60,5

CHAPTER 1

The Aging Man's Survival Guide

INTRODUCTION

Chapter presentations.

Even though the subject of "aging" can be tough for us men to talk about, after reading this book, regardless of whether you read it cover to cover or go directly to specific chapters that attract your interest, I feel confident that you will feel better – even if the experience itself might be a mixed bag of trepidation and appreciation.

But since you've obviously already bought it (thank you again!), I can assume that you are at the very least curious about the topic of male aging and somewhat prepared for the book's facts, explanations, and my very personal accounts.

As mentioned in the preface, my main goal with this book is to provide my fellow men with a deeper understanding of the many changes that the male aging process entails. This so that we can face this stage of life with greater confidence instead of being overwhelmed by what we all will inevitably have to accept and deal with.

As the book covers a wide range of relevant areas within the complexity of male aging, I could argue that it's kind of a guidebook.

While many of my observations and descriptions will be recognizable, I'm certain that some will not correspond at all with the experiences you have. At least not right now. But that's okay. We're all different.

My hope is that after reading this book, it will be easier for you to initiate a discussion among your male buddies (and perhaps even your female friends) and take part of their shared experiences of getting older.

By highlighting many of the psychological, physical, and emotional aspects of male aging, I aspire to destigmatize the aging topic. Encouraging the exchange of encounters and by doing so, gradually demystifying this natural phase of life, should be in everyone's interest, man and woman alike. After all, sharing is caring!

Throughout the book's chapters, you will find several of my personal reflections and anecdotes, at times written with a dash of gallows humor – which has been my way of managing the book's at times gloomy theme.

After reading it, your most valuable takeaway will hopefully be the awareness that you are not alone in tackling male aging. That despite still feeling mentally somewhere between 30 or 35 years old, an age I still identify myself with, you are actually one of all men who sooner or later must go through this quite tumultuous epoch of life.

THE MISSION: ACCEPTANCE

The hardest part of aging, at least for me, has been accepting that I am now an older man. Especially once the symptoms of the process had become so recurring and evident that they could no longer be denied or brushed off as temporary glitches in the machinery.

This is a topic I delve deeply into in the book's epilogue, the chapter aptly named **Dealing with Denial & Mortality**.

Over time, I have realized that there are many ways to slow down and, to some extent, even reverse my biological clock, which I discuss in detail in the chapter **Improving Health & Extending Life**.

In **Brighter Days Ahead**, I have focused on how surprisingly contagious a positive mindset can be, how we can spin almost any difficult situation into something positive and beneficial – and why it's important for us to learn to identify and avoid "Drainers."

While the chapter **Designing Retirement** is reasonably self-explanatory, in **Maintaining Relevance**, I discuss how our identity can be affected when our careers are over and the various ways we can enhance it – including several suggestions for how to increase our importance – within the family, circle of friends, and as part of society.

Navigating Change: Aging & Sexuality is a chapter that describes the natural changes that a man's sexual organs go through and covers both functionality and how to maintain sexual vitality as we age.

By breaking the silence and dispelling misconceptions about this particular subject, my goal has been to provide valuable insights to help us men navigate the changes more confidently and maintain a satisfying sex life even as we age. I suspect this will be one of the book's most read subjects.

The chapter titled **Your Prostate** has most of what you need to know about the prostate, what it does, and more importantly, why this small gland, tucked away somewhere between our bladder and anus, can become a real problem for many men.

You will also read about various examination and diagnostic methods, (including what a PSA test is and why you should have them taken), as well as tips on how to keep the prostate healthier.

If you suffer from persistent health anxiety or even have a diagnosis of hypochondria, you might want to skip **Common Male Illness** and **Big C**. These chapters detail the most common ailments and cancers diagnosed in men aged 55 and older, including the most prevalent type – prostate cancer. Causes, symptoms, and treatments for different types of diseases and cancer are also covered here.

In the chapter **Health Secrecy**, arguably the most important topic of the book is discussed; why we men, especially compared to women, are so pathetically bad at talking and discussing various age-related health problems and diseases that affect us and that we, sooner or later, must acknowledge and deal with.

In the chapter **Invisible Man**, I have turned the spotlight on today's culture, which is so increasingly focused on youth, and how this affects us who are no longer young but still feel capable of contributing significant value to society. This chapter also deals with how many men no longer feel seen and how this can make us feel, act, dress, and talk.

In the books first chapter, **Creaky, Cranky & Confused**, I will guide you through the common physical and mental signs and symptoms of aging. I will also highlight the silver linings and discuss ways to mitigate challenges and avoid significant pitfalls.

Well then. Let's get started.

CHAPTER 2

The Aging Man's Survival Guide

CRANKY, CREAKY & CONFUSED

Tell-tale signs of aging and strategies for how to deal with them.

This chapter focuses on the array of physical and psychological signs and symptoms of aging that can make us feel cranky, creaky, and confused. I have also included several recommendations on how to manage, reduce, and potentially reverse some of these symptoms.

Gentle reader, there is no other way to put this: at some point after reaching middle age, and certainly by the time we've turned 60, we will be facing both permanent and fluctuating signs of our body's inevitable deterioration process.

While you may or may not recognize all of the more or less subtle indicators that follow, the odds are stacked fairly high that sooner rather than later, you will be conscious of some.

Please note that the following collection of manifestations will vary in visibility, strength, and intensity from individual to individual and from age to age. Rest assured that I will also be pointing out the silver linings within this oftentimes sensitive topic.

Okay, let's begin at the top with the more superficial physical attributes of aging…

GRAYING HAIR

This literal silver lining can debut in men as early as when we are in our mid-30s. By the time we reach 50 or 60 at the very latest, most of us won't be able to conceal the onslaught of gray hair without dyeing or bleaching it. But if you're like me, losing most of your mane by the time you had reached 30, this will obviously not be much of an issue.

WHY OUR HAIR GOES GRAY

MELANIN PRODUCTION DECLINES

Hair color is primarily determined by two types of melanin pigments: eumelanin, which is responsible for dark colors (black and brown), and pheomelanin, which is responsible for lighter colors (blonde and red).

As we age, the cells in hair follicles that produce melanin, called melanocytes, gradually produce less melanin. The gradual reduction in melanin production leads to the formation of air bubbles in the hair shaft. These air bubbles scatter light, making the hair appear gray.

GENETICS

Genetics play a significant role in when and how quickly an individual's hair turns gray. If your parents or grandparents experienced premature graying, you may be more likely to do so as well.

ENVIRONMENTAL

Exposure to environmental factors like pollution, smoking, and UV radiation from the sun can contribute to premature graying.

HORMONAL CHANGES

Changes in hormonal levels, like those that occur during male menopause or andropause. Hormonal changes often occur during thyroid disorders which can also influence hair color. Some nutritional deficiencies, particularly deficiencies in vitamin B12 and folic acid, can also be a factor in premature graying.

STRESS

Although the relationship between stress and graying is not entirely understood, chronic stress may play a pivotal role in the premature graying of hair. Hence the saying how parenting can give you gray hair.

HAIR TODAY, GONE TOMORROW.

While many men view baldness as a serious setback, as someone that lost his hair early on, I think it's only fair to point out a few benefits of being bald, both from a practical and a psychological perspective.

CONFIDENCE BOOST

Embracing baldness with a clean-shaven head can boost confidence. At first, this might seem like a somewhat radical step. But it's actually a proactive one that clearly says, "I'm in control of my appearance."

Shaving off your hair can be a way to adapt to change and move forward in a positive way. It signifies your willingness to accept new circumstances and redefine your sense of style. This attitude can have a very positive impact on other aspects of your life, including socially.

A completely shaved head provides a uniform look, eliminating the appearance of thinning or receding hairlines. And if you've been employing the somewhat sad "Robin Hood" comb-over approach, a bald head will provide you with a more honest, neater, and more overall polished appearance.

As your hair continues to thin, it can become increasingly challenging to style it in a way that conceals the loss. Shaving it all off will definitely make it more easily maintained. Also, shaved head is a timeless and classic style that suits a wide range of ages and situations. It can, in my view, project a sense of maturity and sophistication.

The skin of a shaved head breathes better and allows you to more easily apply sunscreen to protect your scalp from sunburn as well as check, should any skin issues arise.

Ultimately, the decision to shave your head, at least when irrevocable hair loss becomes all-too evident, is a personal one. It's about embracing a new look and gaining confidence in your appearance.

Long-term, like me, many of you might find that a shaved head exudes strength, self-assuredness, and a sense of liberation from the constraints of conventional hair beauty standards.

From a maintenance perspective, bald heads are incredibly low-maintenance. No need to worry about bad hair days, styling products, or expensive haircuts. Just a simple wash and you're good to go.

Without the need for expensive and extensive hair care routines, being bald means saving a significant amount of money and time. There are no hassles with dryers, styling tools, or hair products and the natural air conditioning a bald head enjoys helps keep us cooler, especially in hot weather.

WRINKLES

As for everyone, age brings about visible changes in the skin, with facial wrinkles being among the most noticeable signs. These wrinkles occur due to a combination of factors that include the natural aging process, lifestyle choices, and environmental exposure.

As we men age, our skin gradually loses collagen and elastin– proteins that provide the skin with structure and elasticity. This loss, compounded over time, leads to the skin becoming thinner, less hydrated, and more susceptible to sagging and forming lines.

Lifestyle factors like sun exposure, smoking, and poor diet can accelerate this process by breaking down collagen more quickly and damaging the skin. Men's skin, which tends to be thicker and more exposed to environmental elements, may show signs of aging differently than women's.

Facial expressions also play a role; repeated movements like squinting or frowning create wrinkles that eventually settle as permanent features. Keep in mind that the formation of wrinkles is a process influenced by both genetic and environmental factors, which reflects our history of skincare, habits, and life experiences.

DECREASED MUSCLE MASS

Muscles and muscularity, for many a clear sign of strength and masculinity, vigor, and tenacity, will begin decreasing physically and visually by the time most men turn 60. The loss of muscle mass is a process known medically as sarcopenia.

Muscle tissue is metabolically active, meaning it burns more calories at rest than fat tissue. With less muscle, the body's resting metabolic rate (RMR) decreases, leading to a lower metabolism.

There's also a decline in hormone levels, particularly testosterone, which typically occurs as we age and will impact metabolism more or less significantly. Testosterone plays a key role in muscle maintenance and growth.

As levels drop, muscle loss will inevitably increase. This often coincides with a reduced metabolism. In fact, men over the age of 60 often experience a reduction in both the so-called constructive and destructive metabolism processes.

SLOWER METABOLISM

As we get older, our body composition changes with an increase in body fat and a decrease in lean body mass. Since muscle tissue burns more calories than fat tissue, a shift toward higher body fat can also contribute to a slower metabolism.

The constructive metabolism (anabolism) is the process in which your body builds complex molecules from simpler ones, using the energy you've stored in the body. It's responsible for growth, repair, and the synthesis of molecules, including those that make up proteins and DNA.

The destructive metabolism (catabolism) is the process in which the body breaks down complex molecules into simpler ones, releasing energy. It provides the energy needed for various cellular functions and helps remove waste products.

Reduced physical activity, which for most men is on par with aging, will also contribute to our reduced metabolism. There is a wide range of reasons why we stop being as physically active as in younger years, including decreased health conditions, chronic pain, or just a more sedentary lifestyle. Consequently, reduced physical activity leads to a decrease in muscle mass, reduction of calorie expenditure, and a slower metabolism.

Decline in Basal Metabolic Rate (BMR) BMR is the number of calories the body needs to maintain basic functions while at rest. With aging, our BMR tends to decrease due to factors like hormonal changes, loss of muscle tissue, and a general slowdown of many organ functions.

On the upside, a lower BMR also means our body requires fewer calories to sustain itself. So, it's important to keep in mind that as our metabolism tends to slow down with age, we need to maintain a healthy lifestyle that includes regular physical activity of some kind to maintain our overall health and well-being.

CREAKINESS & JOINT STIFFNESS

This common affliction becomes more prevalent as we age. Over the years, my previously agile joints started to feel tight and inflexible, making sounds that accompanied almost every movement, from the simple act of standing to moving about or stretching my arms up.

Stiffness is often the result of the wear and tear of cartilage, the rubber-like padding that covers the ends of bones in a joint, allowing for smooth movement. As cartilage deteriorates, bones might begin to rub against each other, leading to discomfort and a reduction in the range of motion.

Also, the synovial fluid, which serves as a lubricant in the joints, decreases as we age, exacerbating the problem by making the joint movements less smooth and more prone to stiffness and pain.

Obesity, lack of physical activity, and previous joint injuries can accelerate the degeneration of our joint health, making stiffness and pain even worse. Environmental and lifestyle factors, like cold weather and sedentary habits, can also contribute to stiff joints.

Inflammatory conditions like rheumatoid arthritis or osteoarthritis can lead to significant changes in joint structure, thereby increasing stiffness and discomfort. Fortunately, despite all these painful challenges which most of us will experience sooner or later, there are effective strategies to manage, reduce and reverse joint stiffness.

Regular, low-impact exercises like walking, swimming, or yoga can improve flexibility and strengthen the muscles around joints, providing better support and reducing wear and tear. Maintaining a healthy weight also reduces the strain on our joints, especially those of the knees, hips, and spine.

Eating a diet rich in anti-inflammatory foods, including omega-3 fatty acids found in fish and antioxidants in fruits and vegetables, can also help reduce chronic joint pain and stiffness.

Staying clear of hyper-processed foods including most prefab dinners, fast-food meals, power bars, snacks and sugary beverages (natural or artificially-sweetened) will help reduce inflammation by simply improving the health of our gut's microbiome.

Finally, staying hydrated helps maintain the synovial fluid, which can lessen the friction and help keep your joints moving more freely. Warm baths or heat treatments can relax the muscles and reduce stiffness, while cold treatments can reduce swelling and numb the pain. Through a combination of these approaches, it is possible to alleviate some of the discomfort that comes with joint stiffness.

LOSS OF STRENGTH

As I've aged, I have had to come to grips with the sobering reality that my strength, explosiveness, and stamina aren't what they used to be. Feeling my muscles weaken and my energy wane has been daunting, a stark reminder of the relentless march of time. It's disheartening to realize you can't do things with the same vigor as you once did.

Nevertheless, I've learned that this muscle deterioration can actually be slowed down and maybe even reversed. By consciously choosing a healthier lifestyle, increasing and diversifying my exercise regimen, and continually challenging myself physically, Today, I feel like I can retain much of my vitality. I'm not just committed to prolonging my strength, but to also enhancing the quality of my life as I age.

UNBALANCED

My sense of balance has gradually decreased. This is due to a combination of reduced muscle strength, increasingly impaired vision, slower reflexes, and changes in the inner ear that affect my sense of equilibrium.

The decline is normal and began subtly in my early 50s and became more pronounced over time. It's by no means debilitating and mostly rarely something I even think of. Still, it's nevertheless noticeable in certain situations, like if I stumble while taking a step up or down from a curb, walk on uneven ground or when I'm on a slippery sidewalk or surface.

Jumping off of heights, even from or to lower heights, can generate a surprising amount of hesitation and insecurity nowadays. So, to minimize risks and increase my balance, I've become more focused on buying shoes with good support and non-slip soles, as they provide a stable base and reduce the chances of slipping and falling.

I've also adopted a more mindful walking technique and pay closer attention to the surface I'm on as well as making more deliberate, controlled movements.

Regular exercise and balance training, like yoga, Tai Chi, and Qigong have significantly improved my muscle strength, coordination, and proprioception – the body's ability to sense its position in space.

As hard as it is to admit at as early an age as 60 is, I know for a fact that by having a solid strategy in place to reduce the risk of falls and the potentially serious consequences that might ensue, I'm doing what I can to make that I stay healthy and not fall victim to my own carelessness.

EYESIGHT CHANGES

With age, our eyesight unavoidably becomes weaker and there will likely be a need for corrective glasses, like bifocal and/or reading specs. The deterioration can transform once simple tasks, like reading the fine print on medication bottles or a restaurant menu, into pretty frustrating challenges. The once-clear world becomes a bit blurrier, making some precision tasks and detailed work more difficult.

I've become accustomed to using my cellphone's camera to zoom in on small text and always have a small but powerful magnifying glass near my home office desk. These tools allow me to bridge the growing gap between my visual capability and my need to engage with the world around in a clear and undiminished way.

Whatever workaround you choose to use, keep in mind that embracing and overcoming the challenges that come with age will significantly enhance your quality of life, allowing you to continue enjoying favorite reads, menus, and labels without strain or struggle. This also demonstrates a willingness to adapt and resilience in the face of aging.

REDUCED LIBIDO

As I started navigating my 60th year, one of the most interesting yet barely talked about changes among us men, was the slow decrease of my libido. While not entirely diminished, I have noticed a dwindle in my sexual desire and the need to pursue urges that come and go.

I've learned that for men like me in their early sixties, the decline in testosterone level can make sexual desire that once felt like a roaring fire be more akin to a warmly burning ember. I also know now that this is a natural evolution, influenced by a complex interplay of biological factors that cover everything from hormonal changes, health conditions, and the emotional landscape of this chapter in my life.

Interestingly, I've found a richness to this phase of my life, one that I hadn't really anticipated. I have come to see it as an opportunity to rediscover intimacy in ways that transcend sexuality, that deepen my relationship with my wife and which are built on emotional closeness, shared experiences, and an understanding that comes from enduring life's challenges as a team.

While we still have moments of physical, pleasuring intimacy, we can now also find joy in the simple stuff, including the laughter that often fills our home, and the everyday moments shared in each other's presence and together with our daughter – whenever she grants us a visit. Facing this change has also opened the door to conversations about intimacy and desire between the two of us. It's a journey of adaptation, acceptance, and, most importantly, love – a testament to the fact that while certain aspects of our relationship are changing, our commitment to each other remains unwavering.

In confronting the realities of reduced libido at sixty, I've discovered that aging is not only about loss but also about transformation. It's about adapting to change with grace, embracing the present with gratitude, and looking forward to the future with optimism.

URINATION BLUES

Though there are (lucky) men that barely experience any discomfort, the vast majority of us will have to deal with signs and symptoms of aging directly related to urination.

FREQUENCY

As we age, our bladders tend to become less stretchy, reducing its ability to hold urine. This can result in having to pee more often, including a persistent need to wake up multiple times during the night to visit the bathroom.

URGENCY

Some men may experience a sudden and strong urge to urinate, which can be difficult to control. This can lead to situations where you need to find a restroom quickly. This too is within the realm of normal and can be at least partially remedied by budgeting our intake of caffeine, alcohol, and by not drinking excessive amounts of water before going to sleep.

WEAK STREAM

Over time, I've noticed how my stream of urine has become weaker or slower which sometimes makes it challenging to empty the bladder quickly and or completely. While sitting down can certainly be a comfortable way to pee, standing up takes better advantage of the pressure build-up in the bladder and will usually provide me with a shorter visit to the men's room.

INCOMPLETE EMPTYING

It's common for older men to have difficulty completely emptying their bladder, leading to a feeling of not being "finished" after urination.

NOCTURIA

Nocturia refers to the need to urinate frequently during the night. This can disrupt sleep and affect overall well-being. By avoiding drinking (anything) a few hours before going to bed, I can usually reduce my nightly need to pee.

URINE DRIBBLING

After urination, some men may experience dribbling or leaking small amounts of urine, which can be inconvenient. Spending a few extra minutes for those last few droplets can remedy this to a degree.

DIFFICULTY STARTING
Difficulty initiating the flow of urine can be an issue which usually related to prostate enlargement or an infection. It's important to give our bodies the extra time needed in these situations.

PAIN OR DISCOMFORT
Some men may experience pain or discomfort while urinating, which could be related to an infection or other medical condition. In chapters, "Your Prostate" and "This Happens To Your Penis", I'll deal with some of the most common physiological and functional changes that often occur in men with age, including how you'll likely become all-too familiar with your prostate gland.

SKIN CHANGES
As we men approach the age of 60, we can expect some significant changes in our skin. This is entirely driven by decades of environmental exposure, lifestyle choices, natural aging processes, and, of course, genetics.

Our skin may appear thinner, less elastic, and more fragile due to a decrease in collagen production and the gradual breakdown of elastin fibers. This is most often noticed as an increase in wrinkles, age spots, and dryness, as well as a slower rate of cell turnover, leading to a duller complexion.

Sun damage from earlier years may manifest as precancerous growths or skin cancer, underscoring the importance of regular dermatological check-ups. Going forward, staying hydrated, maintaining a healthy diet rich in antioxidants, and avoiding smoking can also mitigate some age-related skin changes and provide us with healthier, more resilient skin in the years to come.

DECREASED BONE DENSITY
For most men 60 and over, a decreased bone density can become a significant health issue, marking an increased risk for fractures and osteoporosis. This decline in bone mass is attributed to lower

levels of testosterone, alongside a deficit of calcium and vitamin D, reduced physical activity, and lifestyle factors.

The thinning of our bones may not have immediate symptoms, but it will eventually heighten the risk for bone fractures, particularly in the hips, spine, and wrists, from falls or even minor stresses.

Weight-lifting exercises, taking calcium and vitamin D through diet or supplements, and undergoing bone density screenings can reduce the impact of decreased bone density and allow you to maintain strength and mobility in later years.

THE AGE OF FATIGUE

I see evidence of it on the streets, among older friends and senior relatives. And then one day, I realize it's even happening to me; a strange and at times debilitating tiredness. I feel sapped, drained, bushed, and completely shattered.

Even getting out of the car, chair, or walking the dog can bring on a disproportionate level of exhaustion that can't easily be related to and that I probably brush off in a nonchalant denial kind of way.

At first, it feels like I just need a longer stretch of road to get going and up to my normal speed. But eventually that road becomes longer and I need even more time to reach my normal cruising speed and agility.

BUT WHY DO WE GET TIRED AS WE AGE?

For me, age-related fatigue became more apparent and tangible as I neared 55. It didn't happen overnight, instead, it was an abstract feeling that crept upon me over a period of several months or maybe even a year. And there was a distinctive correlation between how tired I felt and how I slept, what and how much I drank, the food I ate, and how frequently I exercised.

Regardless though, the reserve of energy I was so used to calling upon whenever I needed to pull an all-nighter, was not nearly as readily available as it once was.

Generally, as part of the natural aging process, fatigue becomes more palpable in our late 50s and early 60s due to a number of factors, including a slower metabolism, hormonal changes (declining production and distribution of testosterone), sleep disturbances, and for many, the influence of a more sedentary lifestyle.

To counter-balance and stave off an increase in fatigue, it's crucial for us to identify limitations but not stop challenging ourselves. Above all, it's important (not to mention life-extending) to prioritize a lifestyle that promotes our physical and mental health. I reduced my fatigue significantly by:

EXERCISING REGULARLY

I aimed for getting at least 30 minutes of moderate-intensity exercise most days of the week. Exercise helped improve my energy levels, reduced mood swings, and improved my sleep quality.

EATING HEALTHIER FOOD

Ever since becoming aware of my metabolism slowing down and seeing how much weight I was putting on, I made a conscious decision to reduce the portions I ate and to eat more food that my now slower metabolism could efficiently turn into useful energy (as opposed to fat).

I've tried to adopt the Japanese phrase "hara hachi bun me" which translates to eating until you are 80% full. Biochemist Clive McCay, a professor at Cornell University in the 1930s, found that a calorie restrictive diet prolonged life in laboratory animals.

INTERMITTENT FASTING

This is a dietary approach where I alternate between eating three meals a day and days where I skip one or two meals and only drink water, coffee or tea in between.

Intermittent fasting is considered logical because historically, our bodies did not evolve to eat three meals a day; food was not always readily available, and early humans often experienced extended periods – days or even weeks – without eating while they hunted and gathered, which suggests that our metabolism is well-adapted to periods of fasting.

Today, we often eat more food than we need, and dining has

become a part of our entertainment-craving lifestyle, leading to overuse of our digestive system. Especially problematic is our consumption of unnatural, processed, and hyper-processed foods, which often require more energy to digest and cleanse than the nourishment they provide.

TWO POPULAR INTERMITTENT FASTING METHODS

16/8 Method: This involves fasting for 16 hours each day and eating all meals within an 8-hour window, commonly practiced by skipping breakfast and eating from noon until 8 PM.

5:2 Diet: This approach involves eating normally for five days of the week while restricting calorie intake to about 500-600 calories on the other two days, which are typically non-consecutive.

Intermittent fasting works well for me, but after I turned 60, with the occasional exception, I also typically choose leaner proteins, reduce the amount of fast carbs and choose nutritious foods that I knew will provide my body with the energy it needs to function properly.

Generally speaking, as we men age, fast carbs, also known as simple or high glycemic index (GI) carbohydrates, should be dodged. Why? Because this type of food is so quickly digested by our body that they often cause a sharp increase in blood sugar levels.

For men over 60, an increase in blood sugar levels is a really bad thing and should be avoided for many reasons, including:

TYPE 2 DIABETES

As we age, our bodies become less efficient at regulating our blood sugar levels. Elevated blood sugar levels, especially if consistently high, are a major risk factor for inviting type 2 diabetes. Diabetes can lead to a slew of other health complications, including heart disease, stroke, kidney problems, nerve damage, and vision issues.

COGNITIVE FUNCTION

Research has shown a connection between high blood sugar levels and cognitive decline in older adults. It may also increase the risk of getting Alzheimer's disease.

NERVE DAMAGE

Elevated blood sugar levels can lead to nerve damage (neuropathy), which can cause pain, numbness, and tingling in the extremities, making it difficult to maintain our balance and mobility.

VISION PROBLEMS

High blood sugar levels can affect the blood vessels in our eyes and increase the risk that we get serious vision problems, including diabetic retinopathy, cataracts, and glaucoma.

IMMUNE FUNCTION

As we age, our immune system weakens, heightening vulnerability to infections, especially when blood sugar levels are high.

WOUND HEALING

Elevated blood sugar levels can slow down the body's ability to heal from wounds and injuries, prolonging rehabilitation and recovery. Getting check-ups regularly and monitoring your blood sugar levels is essential for managing and preventing potential health complications associated with high blood sugar.

Look, if you're already close to or over 60, you're already at a higher risk for all these conditions, and elevated blood sugar levels will likely just exacerbate these risks. Sadly, there is no silver bullet solution.

But you can try mitigating risks by maintaining healthy blood sugar levels through your diet, by exercising regularly, and at all costs avoiding a sedentary lifestyle. Like any flawed human, from time to time, I'll certainly allow myself to indulge in food and drinks I know aren't exactly health-promoting.

But then I remind myself of how short-lived the satisfaction will be and this mindset seems to help stave off temptations that inevitably come my way.

MY LIST OF FOODS AND DRINKS I TRY AVOIDING

White, refined table sugar, sucrose, and high-fructose corn syrup.

HIGHLY PROCESSED WHITE BREAD

I do indulge in polished white rice and dried pasta from time to time. But never the fast cooking kind.

I stopped eating breakfast cereals, especially those with added sugars, when I was about 12 years old.

CANDY AND SWEETS

Sugary soft drinks and fruity, carbonated beverages.

Since flavored waters often contain added sugars and carbohydrates, I'll check the labels for hidden sugars before buying and drinking them.

Most sports drinks are formulated for replenishing carbohydrates and electrolytes during intense physical activity. If I'm not engaged in strenuous exercise, gulping down an energy drink means I'm ingesting unnecessary carbs.

Alcoholic beverages can vary widely in carb content, but all beer and sugary cocktails are high in carbs. Dry wines and clear spirits tend to be lower in carbs.

Milkshakes and smoothies often contain a combination of milk, fruit, and added sweeteners, resulting in a high carbohydrate drink. I prefer my homemade smoothies.

Specialty coffees are often loaded with sugar, syrups, and whipped cream. I opt for plain coffee with minimal add-ons and toppings. With milk alternatives, I choose unsweetened versions to avoid sneakily added sugars. But I have no problem drinking regular dairy milk.

Most fruit juices are laden with added sugars and if not, they are usually processed so much that most health benefits will be negligible.

While I do enjoy natural, raw honey from time to time, even if it is high in sugar and therefore contains fast carbs, I certainly avoid all kinds of fake honey, like "table syrup".

I am extremely weak for real, milk-based gelato as opposed to ice cream which is fundamentally frozen whipped cream and considerably less flavorful (and less nutritious than gelato). Greek or

Turkish yogurt is fine but I avoid brands of yogurt with fruit preserves as they often have added sugars and sweeteners.

I avoid all kinds of cakes, pastries, and most desserts. Unless I'm indulging and have a burger on my plate or tray, I avoid processed potatoes like French fries.

STAY HYDRATED

Drinking enough water is important for health and well-being, including fatigue. I aim to drink the equivalent of eight glasses of water per day. I don't always succeed, but I try hard to keep that goal.

GETTING ENOUGH SLEEP

Most of us need around 7-8 hours of sleep per night. When I'm well-rested, I'm much better able to cope with stress and fatigue and when possible, I enjoy taking a nap sometime after lunch – but not too late in the afternoon. I try to limit caffeine and alcohol. Caffeine and alcohol usually interfere with my sleep, which can lead to fatigue. It's especially good to avoid caffeine and alcohol in the hours leading up to bedtime.

MANAGE STRESS

Stress can contribute to fatigue, so it's important to find healthy ways to manage it. Low-impact stress-reduction can be achieved by going for a long walk, meditating and by practicing Qigong, Tai-Chi and Yoga.

GET REGULAR CHECK-UPS

I strongly suggest you see your doctor for regular check-ups to identify and manage any underlying health conditions that may be contributing to the fatigue you're experiencing. And if you have chronic health conditions like diabetes or heart disease, follow your doctor's recommendations in order to manage your specific illness.

STAY SOCIALLY ACTIVE

Social interaction can help boost mood and reduce feelings of isolation, which can contribute to fatigue. Make an effort to stay connected with friends and family, and participate in social activities that you enjoy.

DAILY LIFE

Moderate exercise. If you're feeling tired, it's important to avoid overexerting yourself. However, moderate exercise can actually help improve energy levels. Engage in activities like gardening or light housework to stay physically active without overtaxing your body.

STAY MENTALLY ACTIVE

Keeping your mind sharp can help to prevent cognitive fatigue. Try activities like chess, puzzles, reading, or learning new skills.

LIMIT SCREEN TIME

Reduce screen time before bed to improve sleep quality by minimizing exposure to blue light from electronic devices.

TAKE SHORT BREAKS

If you have a sedentary job, take short breaks to stretch and move around periodically to combat physical and mental fatigue.

AVOID OVERWORKING

Be mindful of overworking and ensure a healthy work-life balance to prevent burnout.

INDIVIDUAL CONSIDERATIONS

Finally, it's important to note that individual needs and preferences can vary. What works for one person may not work for another. It's important to tailor these strategies to your specific circumstances and consult a healthcare provider for personalized advice on managing fatigue and maintaining good health as you age.

CHAPTER 3

The Aging Man's Survival Guide

INVISIBLE MAN

Navigating shifts in perception.

In what turned out to be this book's most personal and challenging chapter for me to write, I will convey some of my experiences from becoming what I call an "invisible man" and adjusting to a professional world that not too long ago I felt like I was a part of.

Because, despite having a spirit that still has vigor and a mind that continues to thirst for new knowledge and taking on challenges and adventures, the reflection in the mirror, and more poignantly, society's mirror, often tells me a different story.

Sometimes, it feels as if I'm shouting into emptiness, my voice drowned out by the bustling sound of the world moving on without me. I have no problem admitting how this can at times make me feel gloomy and sentimental. The realization that society has subtly, yet effectively, deemed me less relevant because of my age has been a rather large and bitter pill to swallow.

From a rational, evolutionary perspective, I can understand and even relate to society's brutal stamp of irrelevancy. We all have a relatively predetermined shelf-life based on our ability to be productive by contributing biologically as well as financially.

But since defiance has often sparked inspiration and empowered me to take on and overcome challenges, accepting that society now judges my ability to contribute based entirely on my age has been one of my life's toughest trials.

But what is my alternative? To give up, lie down, and just wait for the Grim Reaper to come knocking?

This chapter is largely about confronting ageism. My hope is that by talking more openly about growing older and all that it involves, we men will eventually reduce the topic's stigma until it's so normalized that we reflect less upon age as a measurement of worth and relevance.

I'm questioning the very notions that form opinions about aging. Yes, it's a battle for relevance, recognition, and respect – a fight that, despite difficulties, I am determined to take on – not just for myself, but for every man and woman who has ever felt marginalized by their age.

After all, if the heart and mind refuse to grow old, why should society dictate otherwise?

PERSONAL INVISIBILITY

Both strangers and friends have occasionally remarked that I appear quite youthful for my age. I assume they are suggesting that I'm well-preserved and look a bit younger than I actually am. While I lack concrete proof, my educated guess is that most men receive similar assessments from time to time. *I suspect this might in fact be society's subtle method of softly transitioning us men into what could be considered the Age of Irrelevance.*

There are still episodes, admittedly fewer and fewer, when I'll catch a faint glimpse of my former younger self in a mirror and recall what it was like back in the day when so much in life was smoother (especially my face).

The first signs to emerge arrived unannounced around when I turned 50. These were subtle tell-tale signs, a few crow's feet here and there – mostly in the corners of my eyes.

Like any relatively rational man, I initially tried to see them as signs to a life where joy and laughter had been pursued and enjoyed. I saw the shallow, facial grooves on my face that come naturally with aging as a testament to battles fought, obstacles quashed, and important questions pondered.

The creases on any aging man's face are like receipts from settled debts.

Wrinkles tell stories, not just of surrender to age but also of resilience, of a face that has weathered a few storms and lived to tell the stories, all the while trying to maintain a level of dignity and character.

Aging is not just a mirror of my defeat against the march of time. It's also proof of my triumphs and an exhibition of a life mostly well-lived. In the previous chapter, **Creaky, Cranky, and Confused,** I've detailed more of the typical physical signs and symptoms of male aging, how to adjust, and what you can do to stave off and even reverse them.

THE GENERATION GAP

At some point towards the tail-end of my initial denial phase, just a few months before I was about to turn 60, it became clear to me that I was in fact standing at the doorstep of old age. As I've previously mentioned, I was aware for some time that a transformation was underway. The physical signs and mental indicators had become too evident for me to ignore or fully deny.

But it was when I began observing how less noticeable I was to people younger than myself, especially those in their 20s, 30s, and even 40s, that this realization really dawned upon me on a societal level.

Not only did it seem like younger generations barely saw me, but most also seemed to avoid meeting my eyes as though this would become unbearably awkward. Maybe my all-too-apparent age was reminding them of their parents or grandparents and that by avoiding my eyes, our brief interaction would be quicker and easier to endure. *Perhaps humans are more at ease when communicating with folks their own age?*

At some point, I became hyperaware of the previously somewhat abstract "generation gap". Now it was not only tangible, the fault line was visible and widening rapidly. Worse yet, I realized that I was now on the older side of the divide. Forever young? Not so much.

ATTRACTION

The disconnect between how I saw myself and how the world had come to see me – or rather, chose not to see me, was worrisome. Feeling how my relative appeal, once a reasonably reliable source of confidence as a male, was diminishing. It was being replaced with translucency or invisibility, underscoring my sense of loss and highlighting the transient nature of appearance as a "currency".

As of this writing (2024), I've been a happily married man for over 25 years and have not and do not engage in flirtatious behavior. That said, like most heterosexual men, I find myself looking at women other than my wife, often without even being conscious of it.

Even interacting with women no more than a decade younger than me seemed awkward somehow. The few times I happen to lock onto the eyes of an adult woman, which used to be a pleasant experience without being flirty, it seems to be more of a slip-up, a serendipitous twitch followed by an expression of either embarrassment, or, at worst, vague disgust.

Nowadays, it's usually women my age, 60 and over, who offer me a brief glance or an extended stare. Sometimes, it even extends to a comprehensive top-to-bottom scan which might come across as them sizing me up. While this isn't necessarily surprising or uncomfortable, it's definitely an adjustment.

Sad or pathetic, take your pick, but I sometimes feel caught in an emotional DMZ, a no man's land where I can't help but still feel reflexively attracted to women that are of an age I've long since passed.

For better or worse, this involuntary "radar," which I'm guessing most men have turned on from puberty and onwards, has certainly diminished over time – just not nearly in proportion to my apparent irrelevance to those who l find appealing.

To be clear, I am not saying that I study women to decide whether or not I find them physically attractive, although, just like any average man, that probably does happen, mostly without me even realizing it. I'm pretty sure this "behavior" is biologically instinctive and ingrained in the low-level lines of our genetic code.

PROFESSIONALLY INVISIBLE

The most insidious of prejudices I've encountered so far reared its head in 2022, when I was about to turn 59. The pandemic was finally over and like most folks, I was looking forward to life returning to some kind of normalcy. I assumed that I would bounce back and once more be busy working and getting decently compensated for my efforts.

That never happened.

Instead, as for many people in the creative field, work was not merely scarce, some of my most loyal clients had even replaced me with either in-house talent or younger and presumably less costly creative contractors.

And despite spending many hours filling out upwards of a hundred assignment proposals and applications for indie contractors, most of which I was more than adequately qualified for, I rarely received anything other than an enthusiastic but unmistakably hollow auto-reply from recruiting sites and anemic corporate human resources departments.

At first, the reality of my situation felt downright surreal. It was as if all of my achievements and accolades – which in no small way had come to define my career and the challenges that had propelled me forward – were slowly but surely becoming irrelevant because of my age.

I had relied for decades on my creative ability and my natural capacity to innovate, and execute ideas, to meet and exceed expectations. My efforts were not only recognized but celebrated insofar that I had a remarkable level of client retention and inspiring relationships with most of the contacts at the companies that continuously hired me.

To suddenly find myself on the outskirts of the professional world, watching as opportunities and collaborations that once flowed freely in my direction, albeit not without a normal share of hurdles and hoops to jump through, now bypassing me, was, to put it mildly, jarring.

How could my great track record of completed assignments, satisfied clients, and all accumulated experience and knowledge all of a sudden count for so little?

The shift to the margins of professional relevance forced me to confront uncomfortable truths about the nature of our age-focused society. That those who had once championed my work were now looking elsewhere, favoring the fresh over the familiar, the new over the known, the cheaper over the costly.

The realization that my identity and self-worth had been so closely tied to my professional status was a thorny path to traverse, and the transition from being sought after and a trustworthy creative to someone relegated to the sidelines wasn't just unexpected – it was also somewhat paralyzing.

The glorification of youth is an age-old societal tradition that praises the vibrancy of being young, casting long shadows over those of us in the later stages of life without apology. That my existence felt dimmed by the luminescence of youth isn't merely a casual observation; I'm sure it reflects a tough reality for many men and women.

Realizing that most of my former clients had moved on without me, rendering me invisible to them, was a stark awakening from a life where I believed my contributions, experiences, and talent would hold lasting value until I chose to step back.

This belief, perhaps naive or arrogant, forced me to confront a new reality that I found hard to accept. It wasn't just a shift; it felt like an abrupt extinguishment of the flame that had driven me with passion and purpose, rather than the gentle passing of the torch I had expected.

As I grappled with this transition, the confrontation with ageism was profoundly disorienting. I was indirectly "told" that my time in the sun had passed and that I should gracefully recede into the shadows to make way for a younger generation. This cold comfort made it clear to me: every career, no matter how illustrious, has an expiration date.

That's not to say I wholeheartedly agree with the premise that my relegation was a natural evolution, some kind of reverse rite of passage that all of us, older men and women alike, must simply get over and move on from.

Accepting that my creative ability was to be viewed through a lens tinted with age-based bias and age-related preconceptions generated a stark confrontation with my own mortality.

THE SILVER LINING

Eventually, the resignation and acceptance prompted me to begin a period of introspection and, subsequently, a reevaluation of what reality was telling me; that in my line of creative work, at least at the hands-on production level I had been comfortably operating at (as opposed to pursuing a path of project management and corporate soldiery), age had indeed become a deciding factor.

As I came to terms with this revelation, I began to understand that my value wasn't at all diminished or extinguished by the circumstances in which age had become a factor.

Sure, I might be invisible to the job market. With some hindsight, I can now actually understand why a 60-year-old might not be an optimal fit in a team of vibrant, talented creatives half as old as me.

I started seeing this phase of my life as a new era and an opportunity to rediscover previous creative passions that weren't confined by trivial boundaries like age. One of these rediscovered passions was writing. Hence this book.

AGEISM AND WOMEN

For women, the professional world, already challenging due to gender biases, becomes doubly so under the added weight of age discrimination. This dual pressure can force a lot of women into making decisions about their careers, whether it's stepping down from sought-after positions or feeling compelled to hide signs of aging to remain competitive.

The intersection of sexism and ageism creates a unique predicament for women. While men also face age-related challenges in the workplace, women contend with a societal double standard that often appraises their contributions through the lens of age much more critically. This not only limits their professional opportunities but can also lead to isolation and a sense of devaluation, affecting mental health and overall well-being.

That said, amid these challenges, today, many women are forging new narratives around aging, embracing their years as a badge of honor rather than a mark of decline. They're leveraging their knowledge and experience to mentor, lead, and take on ageist stereotypes and paving the way for future generations.

Addressing ageism, for women and men, requires a cultural shift – a recognition of the value and potential that all individuals, regardless of age, bring to the table. It's a call to action for society, institutions, and individuals to dismantle ageist perceptions and to celebrate the diversity of experience and perspective that enriches our communities and workplaces.

Overcoming Ageism As a creative contractor, I realize that I was at the mercy of my clients and that they were always free to choose a different contractor to supply their creative needs.

As an employee, you should face ageism, address it head-on in a professional manner, ensuring you are aware of your rights and thereby invite a more inclusive workplace where age is irrelevant.

Combating ageism demands a commitment to adaptability as well as to continuous learning. Staying knowledgeable about industry trends, taking relevant courses and going to workshops, and obtaining new certifications will not only underscore your ability to adapt, it also sends a clear message that you're updating your relevance to employers and peers.

Keep in mind that digital tools and platforms continuously evolve and that by updating your proficiency, you will both enhance your competitiveness and dispel myths about how older colleagues, can't keep up with changing times. Networking plays a critical role too; expanding your connections across various age groups and engaging in industry networks can keep you visible and integrated. Mentorship, where you guide younger colleagues can help inspire a culture of learning and mutual respect. Finally, on a personal level, maintaining health and wellness in a vibrant, energetic workplace will help you combat other stereotypes linked to aging.

CHAPTER 4

The Aging Man's Survival Guide

HEALTH SECRECY

Why we men are so silent about our health.

Here, I have focused on why we men mostly refuse to discuss our health concerns, either among ourselves or with women. I find this particularly interesting as it's diametrically different from how women so easily share and exchange their experiences of conditions, illness and diseases within their biological gender.

MENOPAUSE VS ANDROPAUSE

I'd like to start off by noting the fascinating evolution of menopause as a subject and talking point. Once rarely ever discussed (but often joked about, particularly among men), menopause, the natural cessation of menstruation in women typically in their late 40s to early 50s, is now something most women – and some men – are perfectly comfortable discussing even casually.

Menopause signifies the end of fertility, meaning the woman can no longer conceive children, and happens because her ovaries gradually decrease production of estrogen and progesterone, the two hormones that regulate menstruation. The transition to menopause is called perimenopause and can last several years.

During this time, menstrual periods may become irregular but haven't ceased completely. Though menopause is a natural part of aging rather than a medical illness, the hormonal changes and associated symptoms can significantly impact a woman and the quality of her life. Medical treatments and lifestyle adjustments can help manage many menopause symptoms, though not all.

Previously, open conversations about menopause, if they occurred at all, were often treated as something negative – a perspective bolstered by a lack of both knowledge about what menopause was and society's misconceptions about a woman's health and her aging.

IN RECENT YEARS, THERE'S BEEN A SIGNIFICANT SHIFT IN HOW MENOPAUSE IS PERCEIVED IN MOST WESTERN SOCIETIES.

The change in attitude, primarily among men, reflects a broader transformation in attitudes towards women in general, and women's health, as well as a move away from earlier stigmas associated with menopause, fertility, and sexuality. The new paradigm where menopause is an acceptable subject to discuss is thanks to several key societal changes:

OPENNESS, AWARENESS AND EDUCATION

Today, more information is available about menopause, and medical research has demystified many aspects of it. Providing a clearer understanding of the physiological processes involved has made it considerably easier to understand and empathize with the impact menopause can have on a woman's physical, emotional, and mental health.

WOMEN'S HEALTH MOVEMENT

The rise of the women's health movement has also played a crucial role in destigmatizing the perception of menopause. While advocacy has brought attention to the fact that menopause is a natural part of aging, not a disease or a deficiency, the increase in public discussion about menopause, partly due to more open conversations in the media and public figures speaking out about their experiences, has helped normalize and welcomed the subject into both the living room and bedroom.

FOCUS ON QUALITY OF LIFE

There's greater recognition of the importance of quality of life during and after menopause, which has led to more open discussions about managing symptoms, hormone replacement therapy, and lifestyle changes to maintain health and well-being.

CHANGING ATTITUDES

Society's attitudes towards aging, particularly about women, are evolving. Aging is increasingly seen as a process to be embraced rather than shunned, and with it, a more accepting attitude towards menopause.

SEXUAL WELL-BEING

The understanding that women's sexual well-being is important at all stages of life, including post-menopause, has helped normalize discussing the subject. As a result of this, menopause is increasingly viewed not as an end to youth or fertility but as a natural, significant phase in a woman's life.

This more open, positive approach helps women prepare for and manage menopause without having to worry about societal stigma and allow them to instead focus on improving their overall health and quality of life during and after the transition.

THE SILENT MALE

I was recently introduced to the fact that men also go through a version of menopause known as *andropause*. The age-related decline in for example testosterone levels can lead to several symptoms, including fatigue, depression, and both a fluctuation as well as a decrease in men's sex drive.

Similar to how menopause was once mostly perceived as something negative and barely talked openly about, the reluctance of men to discuss andropause or more age specific health concerns, particularly those related to how this phase of life inevitably impacts our body and mind, is usually rooted in societal and cultural norms but also in individual psychological factors.

IN MANY CULTURES, BUT AT VARYING DEGREES, MEN ARE STILL RAISED TO PRIORITIZE TRAITS LIKE STRENGTH, STOICISM, AND SELF-RELIANCE.

Admitting to health problems, especially when related to sensitive parts of the body that could potentially impact sexual prowess and performance, can be seen as a sign of societal invalidation and personal weakness. Shame is clearly a significant factor here.

Admission is not only seen as shameful. It also conflicts with the archetype of the strong, unflinching male. This perceived fragility leads to many men avoiding discussing health and wellness topics altogether.

For example, prostate problems, which might affect urinary and sexual functions, areas closely linked to societal definitions of manhood and potency, can create feelings of shame and embarrassment, or a sense of diminished purpose as a man.

Being diagnosed with prostate cancer or other serious diseases can make many men feel that society's stigmatization of illness, in general, puts a dent in their masculinity – which, in turn, can make them feel a level of vulnerability that is very uncomfortable.

The conception of masculinity and traditional notions of virility – as well as expectations of potency – play a significant part in many men's reluctance to share an illness, even with family and close friends. The dread of being considered less virile or less capable can cause deep insecurity.

When compounded by the privacy and intimacy associated with affected bodily functions like urination, defecation, and sexuality, it's easy to understand why it can be challenging to discuss this openly.

Since sexual capability is still commonly linked to masculinity, even talking about being diagnosed with prostatitis, or, worse yet, prostate cancer, can feel threatening. Either through the physical implications of the disease itself or the side effects from treatment, including erectile dysfunction and reduced sex drive. Beyond these factors, there's also a general tendency among us men to avoid medical consultation or delay seeking help.

BUT WHY?

I think this can be attributed to several underlying reasons. Firstly, there's a cultural and societal expectation for us men to always exhibit strength, independence, and stoicism. Admitting to health issues or concerns, therefore, can be perceived as an admission of vulnerability, which directly conflicts with traditional norms of masculinity.

This pressure can discourage many men from acknowledging health problems, let alone seek help or advice for them. Secondly, there's the fear of the unknown. The possibility of receiving a serious diagnosis can be paralyzing.

Many choose to stay unaware rather than face the reality of a health condition that could potentially change their lives drastically. As we age, the risk of developing chronic diseases and conditions inevitably increases, which is not only challenging to manage but also marks the unavoidable decline that comes with getting older.

By avoiding medical consultations, it's easier to maintain the illusion of health and youth, at least in our own minds. Denial is a normal coping mechanism that allows us to avoid facing the realities of our health and the implications it may have on our lifestyle, independence, and, ultimately, our mortality.

There's also a practical aspect to consider.

The healthcare system can be intimidating, and navigating it can be complex, time-consuming and costly. Concerns about medical costs, lack of time, or skepticism about the effectiveness of medical treatments can also contribute to the delay in getting help.

Financial constraints can be a direct and significant barrier, as men living in poverty often lack adequate health insurance or financial resources to afford medical care. Even in countries with public healthcare systems, there can be costs associated with treatment, including medications, specialized services, or transportation to healthcare facilities.

The fear of incurring medical debt or the inability to afford treatment can deter men from seeking help to proactively, even when they are aware of having serious health concerns.

By normalizing attitudes towards male health issues and encouraging discussions about our well-being openly, we help promote a healthcare environment that is inclusive and responsive to our specific health needs. This can in turn introduce a more proactive approach to health checkups and screenings, particularly for those of us aged 60 and older.

HEALTH ONLINE

Like many others, I too turn to the Internet for a myriad of purposes, including seeking information on health-related topics. Yet all too often, I find myself navigating through a quagmire of questionable content.

Discerning trustworthy sources from a deluge of professionally produced videos and sleek websites, all marketed by a diverse array of hucksters, charlatans, and self-appointed health authorities, can be overwhelming.

For all its potential to disseminate valuable knowledge and information, the web is at the very least equally plagued by misinformation, deceptive claims, and blatant falsehoods, particularly concerning health issues.

Many of these health websites and "health influencers" aggressively push their "groundbreaking" treatments, cures, and wellness solutions, always boasting unmatched results and testimonials galore.

The appeal of online "expertise" is clear, offering the immediate gratification of health advice at our fingertips. The risk arises when we place our health and trust in influencers whose main focus may be on their online popularity and viewer metrics, rather than the validity and dependability of their healthcare "advice."

I've noticed that men, often more so than women, tend to dive deeply into online research. The ease of access to information allows us to rapidly accumulate knowledge and become quasi-experts on virtually any subject.

Whether it's grasping the complex details of World War II submarines or staying updated with the newest tech gadgets, the Internet facilitates this intensive self-learning process with remarkable ease.

But this self-education has a downside, especially when it comes to health-related issues. While researching submarines can be as harmless as it is enriching, using the Internet to diagnose health conditions is always going to be risky.

It's easy to get over-confident about our research skills and believe we can accurately self-diagnose medical conditions based on symptoms we've read about online or through videos watched on platforms like YouTube. But this can quickly become life-threateningly dangerous because it can lead to serious misdiagnosis, delayed medical treatment, or ignoring professional medical advice.

I think it's essential to approach online health guidance with a reasonable dose of skepticism and to understand that the sheen of Internet notoriety is not synonymous with genuine medical qualification.

Getting medical advice from academically educated healthcare professionals, preferably in a clinical setting, can offer a level of assurance and authenticity that simply won't be matched by any faceless or even well-known online personality.

Personally, I've found that direct consultations with medical experts do more than just calm my worries; they steer me towards proven, science-based treatment options, which have so far led me on a path to recovery.

This not only grounds my health decisions in reality but also emphasizes the importance of relying on accredited medical professionals who base their practices on solid research, clinical trials, and a commitment to patient care.

It's important to remember that healthcare professionals undergo rigorous training and must adhere to ethical standards and guidelines that prioritize patient safety and well-being.

The critical distinction between superficial online advice, sometimes fueled by wild hypothesis, the wonders of natural medicine as well as conspiratorial theories about "Big Pharma", and the contrasting depth of knowledge provided by most healthcare professionals, ensures that my health choices are informed, sensible, and ultimately, safe.

I acknowledge that healthcare professionals are not in any way immune to errors, including misdiagnoses and malpractice. These issues are serious and undoubtedly deserve attention and improvement.

However, when comparing professional healthcare facilities with the vast array of online "experts" promoting natural remedies and offering unverified advice for curing various diseases, including cancer, traditional medicine continues to prove – by a wide margin – to be more reliable and credible.

Healthcare professionals' dedication to continuous education ensures they stay informed about advancements and evidence-based practices in their field, a huge difference compared with most online health gurus, whose qualifications, expertise, and motivations are often questionable and may prioritize personal gain over genuine patient health interests.

In this chapter, I've explored some of the main reasons why men are reluctant to discuss health issues, particularly compared to women's openness about their experiences.

By examining the cultural and societal pressures related to male menopause, aka andropause and that they are connected to expectations of masculinity, I've also shed some light on how deep-rooted norms can deter men from seeking necessary medical care.

This discussion underscores the importance of introducing a more open dialogue about men's health in order to help reduce stigma, encourage proactive health behaviors, and improve our overall well-being as we age.

CHAPTER 5

The Aging Man's Survival Guide

COMMON MALE ILLNESS

Recognizing and understanding
health concerns.

This chapter provides a general overview and insight into some of the physical and mental health issues that frequently occur with aging, including their origins, symptoms, treatments, and, where relevant, survival rates.

While the topics may provoke anxiety, it is not my intention to cause panic or fear. Instead, my aim is to share the data and advice that has helped me overcome my own lack of awareness about illnesses and diseases that affect men in their 50s, 60s, and beyond.

It's important to keep in mind that individual experiences with conditions and illnesses can vary significantly and that they are influenced by environmental, genetic, and lifestyle factors.

PHYSICAL ILLNESSES

CARDIOVASCULAR DISEASES

CAUSES: Cardiovascular diseases rank as a top cause of morbidity and mortality globally. Their origins are multifaceted, deeply entrenched in lifestyle choices and physiological changes. The risk escalates with age as the cardiovascular system experiences gradual wear and tear.

Unhealthy dietary habits, characterized by excessive consumption of saturated fats, trans fats, and processed foods, can lead to atherosclerosis, the accumulation of plaque in the arteries. Inadequate physical activity is another key factor; staying active is essential for heart health, aiding in muscle strengthening, blood flow, and the management of weight and blood pressure.

Smoking significantly raises the risk for heart diseases by damaging artery linings and promoting plaque accumulation, thereby increasing the likelihood of heart attacks and strokes.

High blood pressure and elevated cholesterol levels are also pivotal in the onset of heart disease, with both conditions often going unnoticed for years while causing progressive damage to the heart and blood vessels.

Diabetes, especially type 2, also heightens cardiovascular disease risk due to its association with other factors like obesity, elevated blood pressure, and abnormal cholesterol or triglyceride levels.

SYMPTOMS: Symptoms include chest pain or discomfort, often described as pressure, tightness, or squeezing, particularly noticeable during physical exertion or stress. Shortness of breath, palpitations (sensations of a fast, fluttering, or irregular heartbeat), fatigue, dizziness, and fainting spells are also common, indicating the heart's struggle to pump blood efficiently.

In some instances, symptoms might be subtler and could include numbness, weakness, or coldness in the limbs, suggesting narrowed blood vessels. Swelling in the feet, ankles, legs, or abdomen can result from heart failure, where the heart is unable to pump blood effectively.

Not all cardiovascular conditions exhibit noticeable symptoms until advanced stages, highlighting the importance of regular health check-ups for those with high blood pressure, cholesterol, a smoking habit, diabetes, or a family history of heart disease.

Treatments: Managing cardiovascular diseases typically involves a blend of lifestyle modifications, medication, and possibly surgery. Fundamental lifestyle changes include quitting smoking, adopting a heart-healthy diet rich in fruits, vegetables, and whole grains, maintaining regular physical activity, and keeping a healthy weight.

Mitigating stress and managing conditions like high blood pressure, cholesterol, and diabetes are also crucial for cardiovascular health. Depending on the specific condition, doctors may recommend various medications, such as blood thinners to prevent clots, statins to lower cholesterol, beta-blockers to decrease blood pressure, and drugs to regulate heart rhythm or manage heart failure symptoms.

In severe cases, surgical interventions may be required, including angioplasty to open clogged heart arteries or bypass surgery to create a new route for blood flow to the heart. Heart valve repair or replacement might be necessary for valve issues, and in advanced heart failure, complex procedures like a heart transplant may be considered. Treatment plans are highly personalized, based on the type and severity of the disease, as well as the patient's overall health and lifestyle.

Regular follow-ups and treatment adjustments are often needed, underscoring the importance of a collaborative relationship between patients and healthcare providers in managing cardiovascular diseases.

SURVIVAL RATES: Survival rates vary significantly, contingent on the disease's discovery, severity and the effectiveness of treatment.

TYPE 2 DIABETES

CAUSES: Type 2 diabetes in men commonly results from a blend of genetic, lifestyle, and environmental factors. A key contributor is insulin resistance, where the body's cells fail to respond adequately to insulin, a hormone regulating blood sugar. Over time, the pancreas is unable to produce sufficient insulin to maintain normal blood sugar levels, leading to diabetes.

Genetics also plays a role, with a family history of diabetes increasing risk. Ethnicity is also a factor, with certain groups including African Americans, Hispanics, and Native Americans being more susceptible due to genetic, socio-economic, and environmental influences.

Lifestyle choices are significant in the development of Type 2 diabetes. Being overweight or obese, particularly with excess abdominal fat, poses a major risk. A lack of physical activity and poor dietary habits, characterized by high sugar, processed food, and refined carbohydrate consumption, further elevates the risk.

Age is another consideration; risk escalates after age 45, though Type 2 diabetes is increasingly diagnosed in younger individuals due to rising obesity rates. High blood pressure, elevated cholesterol levels, and smoking not only contribute to diabetes development but also heighten the risk of complications.

SYMPTOMS: Type 2 diabetes often manifests with subtle symptoms that may go unnoticed initially. Common signs include increased thirst and frequent urination, as the body attempts to eliminate excess blood sugar. Unusual fatigue or tiredness occurs as cells receive insufficient glucose for energy. Increased hunger signals the body's need for more energy.

Specific symptoms in men, such as erectile dysfunction, can serve as an early warning for poor blood sugar control. Slow-healing sores or frequent infections highlight high blood sugar's impact on the body's healing capabilities. Acanthosis nigricans, characterized by darkened skin in the neck and armpit areas, indicates insulin resistance.

Awareness that these symptoms may develop gradually and may not initially seem alarming is crucial. Early detection and management can prevent or delay diabetes-related complications like heart disease, nerve damage, and vision problems. Men experiencing these symptoms should seek a healthcare provider's evaluation for proper diagnosis and treatment.

TREATMENTS: Managing Type 2 diabetes in men primarily involves lifestyle changes and, when necessary, medication. A healthy lifestyle is foundational, emphasizing a diet low in sugar and refined carbohydrates but high in fiber and whole foods. Regular physical activity significantly improves blood sugar control, with moderate exercises such as brisk walking offering substantial benefits.

Weight management is vital, as excess body fat, especially around the waist, increases insulin resistance. Regular blood sugar monitoring helps men with Type 2 diabetes understand how various foods and activities affect their levels. Quitting smoking, and limiting alcohol are also important for optimal blood sugar control.

When lifestyle adjustments are insufficient to maintain desired blood sugar levels, medications may be prescribed. Metformin, typically the first medication used, enhances the body's insulin sensitivity and reduces liver-produced sugar. Additional medications may be introduced if metformin alone is inadequate, including sulfonylureas to stimulate insulin production and DPP-4 inhibitors for a gentler increase in insulin production and glucose reduction.

In some instances, insulin therapy may be necessary. Regular consultations with healthcare providers are essential to monitor disease progression and adjust treatments accordingly. Awareness and management of associated conditions such as high blood pressure and cholesterol are also crucial to minimize the risk of complications.

SURVIVAL RATES: With appropriate management, Type 2 diabetes can be effectively controlled. However, untreated or poorly managed diabetes can lead to severe physical complications, potentially reducing life expectancy.

ARTHRITIS

CAUSES: Arthritis in men around 60 and older often stems from a combination of age-related wear and tear, lifestyle factors, and genetic predisposition. Osteoarthritis, characterized by the degeneration of joint-protecting cartilage, is prevalent in this demographic, accelerated by years of joint stress and use.

Previous joint injuries, common in physically demanding professions or sports, can predispose individuals to arthritis. Being overweight exacerbates joint pressure, particularly in the hips and knees, hastening cartilage breakdown.

Rheumatoid arthritis, an autoimmune disorder where the immune system attacks joint tissues, can also emerge in older men. Though its exact cause remains elusive, a mix of genetic and environmental factors is suspected. Smoking, especially in genetically susceptible individuals, is a recognized risk factor.

Diet and lifestyle influence other arthritis forms, such as gout, where high alcohol, sugary drink, and purine-rich food consumption (e.g., red meat, seafood) increase risk. Underlying conditions like psoriasis or lupus can trigger various arthritis types.

As age advances, regular health screenings and lifestyle adjustments become imperative to mitigate arthritis risk or delay its onset.

SYMPTOMS: Arthritis symptoms in men, particularly those 60 and older, often include joint pain, described as a consistent ache or discomfort that worsens with movement. Joints may feel stiff, especially in the morning or after periods of inactivity, though stiffness can ease with activity. Swelling in the joints, causing tenderness and warmth, results from inflammation, a hallmark of arthritis.

Aging men might observe a reduced range of motion, making daily tasks challenging. Rheumatoid arthritis can also manifest systemic symptoms, such as fatigue and malaise. As arthritis progresses, joint appearance may change, including the development of knobby finger joints. Symptom severity and frequency can vary, with some men experiencing intermittent issues, while others face continuous challenges.

Consultation with a healthcare provider is essential for men exhibiting these symptoms, as early diagnosis and treatment can significantly improve quality of life and symptom management.

Treatments: Arthritis management in men around 60 and older generally combines medication, lifestyle changes, and potentially surgery to alleviate pain and enhance joint function. Acetaminophen (Tylenol) or non-steroidal anti-inflammatory drugs (NSAIDs) like ibuprofen are commonly employed for pain relief and inflammation reduction. However, long-term use of these medications requires caution due to potential adverse effects.

In autoimmune arthritis types like rheumatoid arthritis, more potent drugs, including corticosteroids or disease-modifying anti-rheumatic drugs (DMARDs), may be necessary to slow disease progression and control immune system activity. Biologics and JAK inhibitors offer targeted treatments for rheumatoid arthritis, focusing on specific immune pathways to manage symptoms and disease course.

Lifestyle modifications are equally important. Engaging in low-impact exercises (e.g., walking, swimming, yoga, qigong, cycling) maintains joint flexibility and muscle strength, with physical therapy aiding in safe exercise planning. Weight management reduces joint strain, especially on weight-bearing joints like knees and hips. Assistive devices (e.g., canes, knee braces) may also relieve joint stress.

For those with advanced arthritis impacting life quality, surgical options, including joint repair, replacement, or fusion, may be considered. Collaborating with healthcare providers to customize a treatment plan addressing specific symptoms and lifestyle factors is crucial for optimal arthritis management.

OSTEOPOROSIS

CAUSES: Osteoporosis in men primarily arises from decreased bone density and strength, an inevitable aspect of a man's aging process. With advancing years, the body's ability to absorb calcium and vitamin D diminishes, while testosterone production, vital for bone density maintenance, declines. This reduction weakens bones, making them more susceptible to osteoporosis. Genetics also influence risk, with a family history of the condition increasing susceptibility.

Lifestyle choices significantly impact osteoporosis development in older men. Inadequate calcium and vitamin D intake accelerates bone loss, while physical inactivity poses a major risk, given the importance of weight-bearing and muscle-strengthening exercises for bone health. Smoking and excessive alcohol consumption detrimentally affect bone health.

Other risk factors include prolonged use of certain medications (e.g., steroids) and chronic conditions (e.g., rheumatoid arthritis, gastrointestinal disorders) that hinder nutrient absorption. Recognizing these risk factors is vital for early intervention and osteoporosis prevention as men age.

SYMPTOMS: Osteoporosis often develops insidiously, with few noticeable symptoms until a fracture occurs. Height reduction and a stooped posture are primary signs, resulting from weakened, compressible spine bones. Bone and joint pain, particularly in the back and hips, may signal osteoporosis. Fractures, especially in the hip, wrist, or spine, often serve as the condition's first apparent symptom, occurring with minimal or no trauma.

Osteoporosis is dubbed a "silent disease" due to the absence of symptoms until significant bone loss or fractures. Therefore, men with risk factors (e.g., family history, smoking history, long-term steroid use) should consider bone density testing for early detection and management, aiming to prevent fractures and preserve bone health.

TREATMENTS: Osteoporosis management focuses on bone strengthening and fracture prevention. Lifestyle modifications are foundational, with adequate calcium and vitamin D intake through diet and supplements crucial for bone health. Weight-bearing exercises and resistance training build bone density and muscle strength, reducing fall and fracture risks. Quitting smoking and moderating alcohol intake are also advised.

Healthcare providers may prescribe medications to enhance bone density and lower fracture risk. Bisphosphonates (e.g., alendronate, zoledronic acid) slow bone loss, while other options like denosumab (administered biannually) and teriparatide (daily injection) stimulate bone formation. Discussing potential benefits and risks of these medications with healthcare providers is crucial, as treatment choices depend on individual circumstances.

Regular follow-ups and bone density monitoring are essential to assess progress and adjust the treatment plan as necessary, ensuring effective osteoporosis management.

CHRONIC OBSTRUCTIVE PULMONARY DISEASE (COPD)

CAUSES: COPD in men around 60 and older mainly results from prolonged exposure to lung irritants. Smoking, the leading risk factor, introduces harmful chemicals that damage lung tissues over time, significantly contributing to COPD development. Secondhand smoke, air pollution, and occupational dust and chemicals also trigger COPD.

Aging naturally diminishes lung tissue elasticity and efficiency in air movement, exacerbating irritant effects. Genetic predispositions may increase susceptibility, while recurrent respiratory infections can cause lung damage, heightening COPD risk. Men with a history of chronic bronchitis or frequent lung infections are particularly vulnerable.

Awareness of these risk factors is crucial for men in this demographic, with smoking cessation and reduced exposure to lung irritants essential for preventing or slowing COPD progression. Early diagnosis and management improve life quality for those with the condition.

SYMPTOMS: COPD in older men manifests with various breathing difficulty symptoms. Chronic coughing, producing mucus or phlegm, is a common sign, often worsening in the morning. Shortness of breath during physical activity or mild exertion may progress to breathlessness during routine tasks, complicating activities like stair climbing or walking.

Wheezing, chest tightness, frequent respiratory infections, and sudden symptom exacerbations are also typical. COPD can lead to unintentional weight loss and fatigue due to increased breathing effort. Recognizing these symptoms is important for early medical intervention, as timely diagnosis and management can decelerate disease progression and enhance quality of life.

TREATMENTS: COPD management involves a multifaceted approach to alleviate symptoms and enhance lung function. Smoking cessation is paramount, directly influencing disease severity and treatment effectiveness. Prescribed medications relieve symptoms and reduce airway inflammation. Bronchodilators relax airway muscles for easier breathing, while inhaled corticosteroids decrease inflammation. Severe cases may require combination inhalers containing both medication types.

Quitting smoking and avoiding lung irritants are critical measures for COPD prevention and symptom reduction. Pulmonary rehabilitation programs, comprising structured exercise and education, improve lung health and breathing. Oxygen therapy benefits those with low blood oxygen levels, and advanced cases might consider surgical options like lung volume reduction or transplantation. Annual flu shots and pneumococcal vaccines are crucial for preventing respiratory infections that exacerbate COPD.

Regular consultations with healthcare providers ensure optimal COPD management, with lifestyle adjustments like a balanced diet and physical activity playing a key role in improving life quality for older men with COPD.

SURVIVAL RATES: COPD prognosis depends on various factors, including disease severity, overall health, and adherence to treatment. While COPD is a progressive condition potentially impacting life expectancy in advanced stages, proper management can significantly improve quality of life and extend lifespan. Smoking cessation and reducing exposure to lung irritants are vital steps.

Collaborating with healthcare providers to develop a personalized treatment plan is essential, as early diagnosis and effective management slow COPD progression and enhance survival rates.

BENIGN PROSTATIC HYPERPLASIA (BPH)

CAUSES: BPH primarily stems from age-related prostate gland changes. Natural prostate enlargement, unrelated to cancer, is a common aging aspect. Hormonal shifts, particularly increased dihydrotestosterone (DHT) levels, stimulate prostate cell multiplication, causing enlargement.

While BPH is prevalent in older men, it does not predict prostate cancer development.

SYMPTOMS: BPH symptoms, resulting from prostate enlargement pressing on the urethra, include increased nighttime urination frequency, disrupting sleep. Urgency, a sudden, hard-to-control urge to urinate, and a weak urine stream, requiring straining to start and stop, are common. Untreated BPH can lead to urinary tract infections or bladder stones, necessitating medical evaluation and treatment consideration for improved urinary function and life quality.

TREATMENTS: BPH management aims to enhance life quality. Mild cases may benefit from lifestyle adjustments like reduced nighttime fluid intake, caffeine and alcohol avoidance, and pelvic floor exercises to strengthen urinary control. Medications relieve symptoms; alpha-blockers ease urination by relaxing prostate and bladder neck muscles, while 5-alpha reductase inhibitors shrink the prostate over time, improving urine flow.

Severe cases or insufficient medication relief may lead to minimally invasive procedures (e.g., transurethral microwave therapy, transurethral resection of the prostate) to remove or reduce obstructing prostate tissue. Rarely, prostate gland removal (prostatectomy) might be necessary. Treatment choice depends on individual symptoms, health, and preferences, warranting discussion with healthcare providers to identify the most suitable BPH management approach.

ERECTILE DYSFUNCTION (ED)

CAUSES: ED arises from physical or psychological factors. Inadequate penile blood flow, resulting from conditions like diabetes, high blood pressure, or atherosclerosis, is a primary physical cause. Nerve damage from diseases like multiple sclerosis or post-prostate surgery can disrupt brain-to-penis signals. Hormonal imbalances, notably low testosterone levels, also contribute to ED, as testosterone is crucial for sexual function.

Psychological factors, including stress, anxiety, and depression, can interfere with erection initiation. Relationship or performance anxiety exacerbates these psychological aspects. Lifestyle choices, such as excessive alcohol, smoking, and drug use, further contribute to ED by affecting overall health and blood flow.

Recognizing that ED often involves both physical and psychological factors is key to effective treatment. Healthcare provider consultation can help identify underlying causes and determine the most suitable treatment approach.

SYMPTOMS: ED challenges include difficulty achieving or maintaining a firm erection for satisfactory sexual activity, reduced sexual desire, and emotional or psychological distress related to sexual performance. Occasional erection issues are common, but persistent problems warrant healthcare provider evaluation for diagnosis and treatment options.

TREATMENTS: ED management offers various options, including oral medications (e.g., sildenafil, tadalafil, vardenafil) to increase penile blood flow, facilitating erection achievement and maintenance when aroused. Alternatives for those unresponsive to oral medications include vacuum erection devices, penile injections, and surgically implanted penile implants.

Lifestyle modifications, such as a balanced diet, regular exercise, and stress reduction, can improve ED. Counseling or therapy may benefit men with psychological ED contributors. Consulting with healthcare providers is essential to identify the most appropriate treatment based on individual needs and preferences.

MENTAL ILLNESSES

DEPRESSION

CAUSES: Depression in men aged 60 and older results from a mix of physical, psychological, and life-related factors. Aging-related brain chemistry and hormone level changes can affect mood regulation and heighten depression risk. Chronic illnesses or pain contribute to depression by increasing stress and reducing life quality.

Psychological factors, including mental health history or significant personal losses (e.g., loved one's death, retirement, financial stress), can lead to depression. Social isolation, more prevalent in older age, exacerbates feelings of loneliness and sadness. Recognizing that depression in older men stems from various factors is crucial, with professional help and loved one support essential for managing the condition effectively.

SYMPTOMS: Depression manifestations vary, with many older men experiencing symptoms beyond sadness, such as a significant loss of interest in previously enjoyed activities, social withdrawal, sleep disturbances, appetite and weight changes, physical symptom complaints (e.g., aches, pains), concentration and memory issues, and emotional distress.

Recognizing these symptoms is vital for seeking professional help, as depression is treatable, significantly improving overall well-being.

TREATMENTS: Depression management typically involves psychotherapy (e.g., cognitive-behavioral therapy), medications (e.g., antidepressants), and lifestyle changes. Research into cannabis and magic mushrooms (psilocybin) micro-dosing for depression treatment is ongoing, with potential therapeutic benefits under investigation. Consulting healthcare providers is crucial before considering alternative treatments, ensuring established treatment options exploration and understanding potential risks and benefits.

Survival Rates: Depression in older men poses a significant suicide risk, with many hesitant to express emotional distress, complicating loved one recognition of their suffering. Social isolation, chronic health issues, and significant life changes can exacerbate feelings of hopelessness. Friends, family, and healthcare providers play key roles in depression recognition and treatment, reducing suicide risk and improving older men's mental health.

ANXIETY DISORDERS

CAUSES: Anxiety disorders in men over 60 stem from a blend of physical health, life experience, and emotional factors. Aging-related conditions (e.g., heart disease, diabetes, neurological disorders) can trigger or worsen anxiety. Medication side effects and lifestyle choices (e.g., smoking, alcohol) also contribute to anxiety.

Significant life changes, including retirement and loved one loss, can fuel anxiety, with mental health stigma and a lack of social support compounding the issue. Recognizing these factors is important for understanding and addressing anxiety disorders in this demographic.

SYMPTOMS: Anxiety manifests through psychological symptoms (e.g., excessive worry, restlessness, concentration difficulties) and physical symptoms (e.g., muscle tension, headaches, rapid heartbeat), often mistaken for other medical conditions. Recognizing these symptoms is crucial for seeking appropriate evaluation and treatment.

TREATMENTS: Anxiety disorder management involves psychotherapy, medication, and lifestyle changes, with cognitive-behavioral therapy proving highly effective. Medications (e.g., antidepressants, anti-anxiety drugs) require careful consideration in older patients due to potential side effects. Lifestyle adjustments, such as exercise, diet, sleep, and stress management techniques, significantly help symptom management.

Recent interest in micro-dosing cannabis and magic mushrooms (psilocybin) for anxiety treatment warrants careful consideration, with ongoing research into their efficacy and safety. Consulting healthcare professionals is essential for exploring all treatment options and ensuring legal and medical guideline compliance.

Cognitive Decline and Dementia (Including Alzheimer's Disease)

CAUSES: Cognitive decline and dementia result from genetic, environmental, and lifestyle factors. Genetics increase risk, while aging remains the most significant factor. Other contributors include head trauma, cardiovascular issues, and lifestyle choices (e.g., physical inactivity, poor diet, smoking, alcohol).

SYMPTOMS: Initial symptoms often include memory loss, difficulty planning or solving problems, language issues, visual and spatial relationship struggles, mood and personality changes, and advanced-stage physical ability and behavior alterations. Symptoms vary and progress differently for each individual.

TREATMENTS: Managing cognitive decline and dementia focuses on symptom management and quality of life maintenance, with medications (e.g., cholinesterase inhibitors, memantine) commonly used. Non-medical interventions, such as mentally stimulating activities, social connections, regular exercise, and a structured routine, are crucial. Emerging interest in micro-dosing cannabis and magic mushrooms (psilocybin) for treatment requires careful consideration, emphasizing consultation with healthcare professionals to understand potential risks and benefits.

SLEEP DISORDERS (INCLUDING SLEEP APNEA)

CAUSES: Sleep disorders in men over 60 are linked to physical health changes, lifestyle factors, and aging-related alterations in sleep architecture and melatonin production. Sleep apnea risk factors include increased fatty deposits around the upper airway, overweight or obesity, and lifestyle choices (e.g., smoking, alcohol). Medications and other health conditions (e.g., chronic pain, diabetes, heart disease) also disrupt sleep.

SYMPTOMS: Common sleep disorder symptoms include loud, chronic snoring, frequent awakenings, daytime sleepiness, difficulty concentrating, and decreased libido. Other manifestations include difficulty falling or staying asleep (insomnia) and restless legs syndrome. Changing sleep patterns with age lead to earlier bedtimes, wake times, and lighter sleep.

TREATMENTS: Sleep disorder management involves lifestyle changes, medical devices (e.g., CPAP machine for sleep apnea), and sometimes medication. Good sleep hygiene, establishing a regular sleep schedule, and cognitive-behavioral therapy for insomnia are effective strategies. Medications for sleep aid are generally recommended for short-term use due to potential side effects, especially in older men.

Collaborating with healthcare providers ensures the most suitable treatment based on the specific type and severity of the sleep disorder, aiming to improve sleep quality and overall quality of life.

I hope this chapter has shed light on some of the most common illnesses and diseases men may encounter as we age, from cardiovascular issues to cognitive decline. Writing it has certainly been an enlightening experience for me, and I trust it has empowered you as well.

By taking proactive steps to regularly monitor our health and recognize symptoms early, we can potentially improve our well-being in the years ahead and possibly even extend our life.

CHAPTER 6

The Aging Man's Survival Guide

THE BIG C

Causes, symptoms, treatments.

While the outlook for research and treatment is continuously evolving, cancer has been around for a long time. This chapter covers significant periods in cancer history, the most common types of cancer diagnosed in men aged 50 and older, their causes, treatments, and survival statistics.

There's also a section about emerging technologies that could potentially have an impact on the future of cancer diagnosis and treatments.

Please keep in mind that this chapter is an overview based on my findings at the time of writing it. As the field of cancer research is rapidly evolving, I encourage you to seek the latest information from reliable sources regularly.

CANCER HISTORY

Although the scientific understanding of cancer has advanced significantly over the centuries, historically, the recognition of it as a disease dates back several millennia. The earliest recorded cases of cancer can be found in ancient Egyptian and Greek texts.

The earliest known descriptions of cancer appear in the Edwin Smith Papyrus, an ancient Egyptian text dating back to around 1600 BC, also known as 'The Secret Book of the Physician.

The text describes several cases of tumors or ulcers of the breast that were treated by "cauterization," or burning of the skin in the related treatment area, with a tool called the "fire drill."

The Greek physician Hippocrates, often referred to as the 'Father of Medicine,' was the first to use the terms 'carcinoma' and 'carcinos' to describe non-ulcer forming and ulcer-forming tumors. These terms were derived from the Greek word for crab, "karkinos," possibly because the finger-like spreading projections from cancer reminded him of the shape of a crab.

Another Greek physician, Galen, used the word "oncos" (Greek for swelling) to describe tumors. His beliefs and teachings about cancer were the basis of medical knowledge for centuries in Europe.

18TH TO 19TH CENTURIES

There was significant progress in the understanding of cancer in the 18th and 19th centuries. Surgeons like John Hunter (1728–1793) suggested that some cancers could be cured by surgery, and new techniques in microscopy in the 19th century allowed scientists to look at cancer cells for the first time, leading to advancements in cancer research.

20TH CENTURY ONWARDS

Significant breakthroughs in understanding the biology, genetics, and causes of cancer have primarily happened in the 20th and 21st centuries. The discovery of oncogenes, tumor suppressor genes, and the role of DNA mutations in cancer development were pivotal in understanding how cancer evolves and spreads.

As a concept, cancer has been recognized for thousands of years. But it is only in recent history that a deeper understanding of mechanisms, causes, and treatments has been developed.

TYPES OF CANCER

Cancer is a leading cause of death globally, and its prevalence increases with age.

I've compiled a list of the most common types of cancer diagnosed in men 50 years and older, along with causes, symptoms, treatments, survival statistics, and, where applicable, life expectancy for the most lethal cases.

PROSTATE CANCER

According to research, a large proportion of men – between 60 and 80% – are likely to develop some form of prostate cancer by the age of 80. However, while many may show microscopic signs of prostate cancer as they reach an older age, the percentage who are diagnosed with clinically significant prostate cancer, which requires treatment, is considerably lower.

In the chapter **Your Prostate** I've covered some of the more detailed aspects of having your prostate examined by a healthcare professional – including what to expect from various examination procedures.

According to the US government's Center for Disease Control, all men are at risk for getting prostate cancer. Regardless of ethnicity and social standing.

Out of every 100 American men, regardless of race, about 13 will get prostate cancer during their lifetime, and about 2 to 3 of those men will die from it.

According to research from Sweden's Medical University, Karolinska Institute, every year around 10,000 men in Sweden receive the diagnosis of prostate cancer, and the percentage of Swedish men who die from the disease within five years is about 5%.

This makes prostate cancer the most common and deadliest form of cancer for Swedish men. Breast cancer is the most common form of cancer for Swedish women and lung cancer is the deadliest. Researchers are struggling to find ways of preventing prostate cancer, but so far, there is only guidance for how to minimize risk through lifestyle choices.

Getting your prostate checked regularly after turning 60 is very important as prostate cancer can be treated with various methods, depending on the stage of the cancer, age and overall health – as well as other individual health factors.

CAUSES: Exactly why men get prostate cancer is not fully understood. But several key factors have been identified that increase the risk of developing the disease. Age is the most significant risk factor, with the likelihood of prostate cancer increasing significantly after the age of 50.

A family history of prostate cancer also elevates the risk, suggesting a genetic component to the disease. Certain ethnicities, particularly African American men, have higher rates of prostate cancer, indicating that genetics and possibly environmental factors play a role. Additionally, diet is believed to influence the risk of developing prostate cancer.

A diet high in red meat and saturated fat and low in fruits and vegetables have been linked to prostate cancer, though the exact mechanism is still being researched.

SYMPTOMS: Difficulty urinating, including a weak or interrupted urine flow, is one of the most common symptoms. This occurs as the enlarging prostate gland presses on the urethra, affecting urine flow. Blood in the urine (hematuria) is another alarming symptom that warrants medical attention, as it can be a sign of prostate cancer or other medical conditions.

Additionally, persistent pelvic pain or discomfort in the lower back, hips, or thighs can be symptomatic of advanced prostate cancer, indicating that the cancer may have spread beyond the prostate gland. It's important for men experiencing these symptoms to seek medical evaluation to determine the cause and appropriate treatment.

TREATMENTS: Active surveillance, surgery, radiation therapy, hormone therapy.

ACTIVE SURVEILLANCE OR WATCHFUL WAITING

For very early-stage prostate cancer or in older patients with less aggressive cancer, doctors might suggest monitoring the cancer closely and only treating it if it shows signs of getting worse.

SURGERY

Radical prostatectomy, the removal of the entire prostate gland and some surrounding tissue, is a common surgical treatment. This can be done through open surgery or laparoscopically, often with robotic assistance.

RADIATION THERAPY

This method uses high-energy rays or particles to kill cancer cells. It can be delivered externally (external beam radiation) or internally (brachytherapy, where radioactive seeds are placed directly in or near the tumor).

HORMONE THERAPY

Prostate cancer cells often need male hormones to grow. Hormone therapy reduces the body's production of these hormones or blocks their effect on cancer cells. This is also called androgen deprivation therapy (ADT).

CHEMOTHERAPY

By using drugs to kill rapidly growing cells, including cancer cells, chemotherapy might be the preferred treatment if prostate cancer has spread outside the prostate gland and hormone therapy isn't working.

IMMUNOTHERAPY

This involves using medicines to help the patient's immune system recognize and destroy cancer cells more effectively. Sipuleucel-T (Provenge) is an example of an immunotherapy used in prostate cancer.

TARGETED THERAPY

Targeted drugs can block specific abnormalities present in cancer cells. For prostate cancer, PARP inhibitors are an example of targeted therapy used particularly in men with mutations in certain genes like BRCA1 or BRCA2.

CRYOTHERAPY

Cryotherapy kills cancer cells by freezing them. It's less commonly used and might be an option for treating early-stage prostate cancer in certain cases.

HIGH-INTENSITY FOCUSED ULTRASOUND (HIFU)

This treatment uses high-frequency ultrasound energy to heat and destroy cancer cells in the prostate.

BONE-DIRECTED TREATMENT

For prostate cancer that has spread to the bone, treatments like bisphosphonates and denosumab can help manage bone pain and other symptoms.

The choice of treatment depends on many factors, including how fast the cancer is growing, how much it has spread, the potential side effects of the treatment, and the patient's preferences and overall health. It's crucial for anyone diagnosed with prostate cancer to discuss their treatment options with their healthcare team to determine the best approach for their individual situation.

SURVIVAL STATISTICS: 5-year survival rate is about 98%.

LIFE EXPECTANCY: Generally favorable; varies based on stage and response to treatment.

LUNG CANCER

CAUSES: Smoking is the leading cause of lung cancer in men, which includes cigarettes, cigars, and pipe tobacco. Tobacco smoke contains carcinogens that damage lung cells. Over time, the damage can lead to cancer, with the risk increasing with the number of years and amount of tobacco smoked.

Non-smokers exposed to secondhand smoke at home or work also face an expanded threat of lung cancer. Inhaling the smoke from others carries many of the same risks as smoking itself, due to the harmful carcinogens present.

Radon is a naturally occurring radioactive gas that results from the breakdown of uranium in soil and rocks. It can seep into buildings and accumulate to high levels, leading to a higher probability of getting lung cancer, particularly in homes with poor ventilation.

Certain occupations that involve exposure to carcinogens like asbestos, arsenic, diesel exhaust, and some forms of silica and chromium are at a higher risk for developing lung cancer. Protective measures and regulations are essential to minimize exposure in these work environments.

SYMPTOMS: A cough that does not go away over time and may worsen can be a sign of lung cancer. It is one of the earliest and most common symptoms. Coughing blood can range from a small amount of blood in the saliva and mucus (sputum) to more significant bleeding and is a symptom that warrants immediate medical attention.

Lung cancer can also cause pain in the chest, shoulder, or back area, which might be sharp, dull, or intermittent. It may occur with deep breathing, coughing, or laughing. Lung cancer can also be manifested in a feeling of being winded or short of breath. This symptom may occur if cancer grows to block the major airways or if fluid starts to collect around the lungs.

TREATMENTS

SURGERY

For patients with early-stage lung cancer, surgery may offer a chance to remove the tumor entirely. Types of surgery include lobectomy, segmentectomy, wedge resection, and pneumonectomy, depending on the tumor's size and location.

CHEMOTHERAPY

This treatment uses drugs to kill cancer cells or stop them from growing and dividing. Chemotherapy can be used before surgery to shrink tumors, after surgery to kill any remaining cancer cells, or as the main treatment for those who cannot undergo surgery.

RADIATION THERAPY

This treatment uses high-energy rays to target and kill cancer cells. It is often used in combination with chemotherapy, especially for patients who cannot undergo surgery, and can also be used to alleviate symptoms of advanced lung cancer.

TARGETED THERAPY

This newer form of treatment targets specific genes, proteins, or the tissue environment that contributes to cancer growth and survival. This approach can be more effective and less harmful to normal cells compared to chemotherapy and is usually used for advanced stages of lung cancer with specific genetic mutations.

SURVIVAL STATISTICS: 5-YEAR SURVIVAL RATE IS ABOUT 19% OVERALL.

LIFE EXPECTANCY: Median survival time for advanced lung cancer is less than 1 year; with treatment, 2-5 years depending on which stage.

COLORECTAL CANCER

CAUSES: The risk of developing colorectal cancer increases significantly with age, particularly after 50 and is one of the primary risk factors due to the cumulative effects of lifestyle and genetic factors over time.

Diets high in fat, especially from animal sources, have been associated with a greater risk of colorectal cancer. These diets may also be low in fiber, which is believed to play a protective role against the development of colorectal cancer.

Having a family history of colorectal cancer or colorectal polyps increases an individual's risk. This risk is apparently higher if the relative was diagnosed with colorectal cancer at a younger age or if multiple first-degree relatives are affected.

Conditions such as Crohn's disease and ulcerative colitis also increase the risk of colorectal cancer due to chronic inflammation in the colon.

Smoking tobacco is linked to an increased risk of developing colorectal cancer. The harmful substances in tobacco smoke can lead to genetic mutations in the colon and rectum, contributing to cancer development.

SYMPTOMS: The presence of bright red or very dark blood in the stool can be a sign of colorectal cancer. This symptom should prompt an immediate consultation with a healthcare provider. Constipation, diarrhea, or a change in the consistency of stool that lasts for more than a few days can also signal colorectal cancer.

Persistent abdominal pain or discomfort, including cramps, gas, or pain that may come with a feeling of the bowel not completely emptying, can be symptoms of colorectal cancer.

TREATMENTS

SURGERY

The main treatment for colorectal cancer, especially in its early stages, involves surgical removal of the tumor and surrounding tissue. The type of surgery depends on the tumor's location, size, and cancer stage. Techniques range from minimally invasive procedures, like polypectomy and laparoscopy, to more extensive surgeries, like colectomy.

CHEMOTHERAPY

Used before or after surgery, chemotherapy involves using drugs to destroy cancer cells. It can help reduce the risk of cancer recurrence and is also used to treat advanced colorectal cancer by shrinking tumors and relieving symptoms.

RADIATION THERAPY

This treatment uses high-energy rays to target and kill cancer cells. It's often used in combination with chemotherapy before surgery to shrink tumors, making them easier to remove. It can also be used to relieve symptoms in advanced colorectal cancer cases.

SURVIVAL STATISTICS: 5-YEAR SURVIVAL RATE IS ABOUT 64%.

LIFE EXPECTANCY: Varies – early detection significantly improves outcomes.

BLADDER CANCER

CAUSES: Smoking is the single greatest risk factor for bladder cancer in men. Harmful chemicals in tobacco smoke are processed by the bladder during urine production, which can lead to cellular damage and increase cancer risk.

Occupational exposure to certain industrial chemicals used in dye, rubber, leather, textiles, and paint manufacturing significantly increases the risk of developing bladder cancer. These chemicals, when processed by the body, may cause harmful mutations in the bladder's cells.

Recurrent urinary tract infections (UTIs), bladder stones, and other conditions causing prolonged bladder inflammation can increase the risk of bladder cancer. Chronic inflammation might lead to changes in the bladder cells, potentially leading to cancer.

SYMPTOMS: The most common and often earliest sign of bladder cancer is blood in the urine (hematuria), which may be visible to the eye or detectable only under a microscope. An increased need to urinate more often than usual can be a symptom of bladder cancer, although this is also common in many other conditions.

Pain or discomfort in the lower abdomen or pelvic area can indicate advanced bladder cancer or growths large enough to press against other structures in the pelvis.

TREATMENTS

SURGERY

Surgery is a common treatment for bladder cancer, ranging from transurethral resection of bladder tumor (TURBT) for early-stage cancers to more invasive options like a radical cystectomy, which involves the removal of the bladder and surrounding tissues, for more advanced cases.

CHEMOTHERAPY

Chemotherapy can be administered directly into the bladder (intravesical chemotherapy) for early-stage cancer or systemically to treat advanced cancer. It works by killing cancer cells or stopping them from dividing.

IMMUNOTHERAPY

This treatment option uses the body's immune system to fight cancer. Bacillus Calmette-Guérin (BCG) therapy, a form of intravesical immunotherapy, is often used for non-muscle-invasive bladder cancer. Systemic immunotherapies that target specific pathways cancer cells use to avoid immune system detection are also used for advanced bladder cancer.

RADIATION THERAPY

Radiation therapy may be used as a primary treatment for bladder cancer, especially for patients who cannot undergo surgery, or in combination with chemotherapy to enhance its effectiveness. It involves using high-energy beams to target and kill cancer cells.

SURVIVAL STATISTICS: 5-YEAR SURVIVAL RATE IS ABOUT 77%.

LIFE EXPECTANCY: Generally good with early diagnosis and treatment.

MELANOMA (SKIN CANCER)

CAUSES: The primary cause of melanoma is exposure to ultraviolet (UV) radiation from the sun. UV rays damage the DNA in skin cells, leading to mutations that can result in melanoma. Both men and women who spend a lot of time outdoors without proper sun protection are literally magnifying the risk of getting melanoma.

The use of tanning beds, which emit UV rays, significantly increases the risk of developing melanoma. These artificial sources of UV radiation can be even more intense than sunlight, leading to greater damage in a shorter amount of time.

A family history of melanoma or inherited genetic mutations increases the risk of developing skin cancer. Certain genes that can be passed down through families make individuals more susceptible to the effects of UV radiation on their skin.

SYMPTOMS: One of the most noticeable signs of melanoma is the appearance of new moles or changes in existing moles. Changes may include alterations in size, shape, color, or texture. Moles that are asymmetrical, have irregular borders, or multiple colors should be evaluated by a healthcare provider.

In addition to moles, melanoma can manifest as new growths or lesions on the skin. These can appear suddenly and may grow or change rapidly. Any new, unusual, or rapidly changing growths should be examined by a professional.

TREATMENTS

SURGERY

The primary treatment for early-stage melanoma is surgical removal of the tumor and a margin of healthy tissue to ensure all cancerous cells are removed. For more advanced melanoma, surgery may involve removing nearby lymph nodes to prevent spread.

CHEMOTHERAPY

While less commonly used for melanoma than other cancers, chemotherapy can be an option, especially for advanced cases. It involves using drugs to kill cancer cells or stop their growth, but it may not be as effective as other treatments for melanoma.

RADIATION THERAPY

Radiation therapy may be used to destroy melanoma cells, particularly in areas where surgery is difficult or to relieve symptoms of advanced melanoma. It's also used to treat melanoma that has spread to the brain or other parts of the body.

IMMUNOTHERAPY

Immunotherapy treatments boost the body's immune system to better fight the melanoma. Drugs like checkpoint inhibitors or cytokines help the immune system recognize and attack cancer cells more effectively. Immunotherapy has become a key treatment for advanced melanoma, offering significant benefits for many patients.

Survival Statistics: 5-year survival rate is about 93% for localized melanoma.

LIFE EXPECTANCY: Varies; early detection greatly improves prognosis.

NON-HODGKIN LYMPHOMA

CAUSES: The risk of developing non-Hodgkin lymphoma increases with age, with a higher incidence in men over 60 years. Aging can lead to changes in the lymphatic system that may contribute to the development of this cancer. Men with compromised immune systems, either from inherited conditions, medical treatments like organ transplants, or diseases such as HIV/AIDS, have a heightened risk of developing non-Hodgkin lymphoma due to reduced capability to fight off cancerous changes.

Infections with specific viruses and bacteria, including Epstein-Barr virus (EBV), Human T-cell lymphotropic virus (HTLV), and Helicobacter pylori, have been linked to an increased risk of certain types of non-Hodgkin lymphoma. These infections can cause chronic inflammation or directly affect the DNA of lymphocytes, leading to cancer.

Having a close relative with non-Hodgkin lymphoma or other lymphatic cancers slightly increases the risk. This suggests a genetic predisposition to the disease, although specific inherited genetic mutations have not been widely identified.

SYMPTOMS: One of the most common signs is painless swelling of lymph nodes in the neck, armpits, or groin. This swelling is caused by the accumulation of cancerous lymphocytes in the lymphatic system.

Persistent fatigue that does not improve with rest can be a symptom of non-Hodgkin lymphoma, often resulting from the body's response to the cancer.

Unexplained fevers, especially when they occur without an identifiable infection, can be a sign of non-Hodgkin lymphoma. The fever may come and go and is usually higher in the evening.

Unintentional weight loss of 10% or more of body weight over six months or less without trying is another symptom. This occurs as the body's metabolism speeds up to fight the cancer.

TREATMENTS

CHEMOTHERAPY

The use of drugs to kill cancer cells is a common treatment for non-Hodgkin lymphoma. Chemotherapy can be administered orally or through intravenous infusion and is often combined with other treatments for better effectiveness.

RADIATION THERAPY

This treatment uses high-energy radiation to target and destroy cancer cells, usually in a specific area. Radiation therapy can be used for early-stage non-Hodgkin lymphoma or to relieve symptoms in more advanced stages.

STEM CELL TRANSPLANT

After high doses of chemotherapy and/or radiation therapy to destroy the cancerous cells, stem cell transplants can be used to restore the body's ability to produce healthy blood cells. This treatment is usually considered for aggressive or relapsed non-Hodgkin lymphoma.

IMMUNOTHERAPY

These treatments help the immune system recognize and attack cancer cells. For non-Hodgkin lymphoma, monoclonal antibodies, checkpoint inhibitors, and CAR-T cell therapy are types of immunotherapy that can be used based on the specific characteristics of the cancer. Immunotherapy is increasingly becoming a key component of treatment strategies, offering new hope for patients with certain types of non-Hodgkin lymphoma.

SURVIVAL STATISTICS: 5-year survival rate is about 72%.

LIFE EXPECTANCY: Varies widely depending on subtype and stage.

KIDNEY CANCER

CAUSES: Smoking tobacco doubles the risk of kidney cancer in men as it contains harmful chemicals that can cause mutations in kidney cells, leading to cancer. Excess body weight, taking certain medications and long-term dialysis is also strongly linked to a raised probability of developing kidney cancer. Fat tissue can produce hormones that may promote cancerous growth in the kidneys.

Hypertension, or high blood pressure, can damage the kidneys over time and has been associated with a higher risk of kidney cancer. The exact mechanism is not fully understood but may involve changes in hormone levels and kidney function.

A family history of kidney cancer also increases the risk. This can be due to inherited genetic mutations that make a person more susceptible to developing the disease.

SYMPTOMS: The presence of blood in the urine, known as hematuria, is a common and often early symptom of kidney cancer. The blood may be visible to the naked eye or detectable only under a microscope. Pain on one side of the back, below the ribs but not caused by injury, can be a symptom of kidney cancer. The pain is usually persistent and can range from mild to severe.

Unexplained weight loss, not related to diet or exercise, can indicate kidney cancer. This symptom often occurs in the later stages of the disease and may accompany a general feeling of being unwell.

TREATMENTS

SURGERY

The primary treatment for localized kidney cancer is surgery to remove the tumor. Depending on the size and location of the tumor, surgery may involve removing the entire kidney (nephrectomy) or just the tumor and a small margin of healthy tissue around it (partial nephrectomy).

TARGETED THERAPY

These drugs specifically target molecular pathways involved in the growth and spread of cancer cells, sparing normal cells. Targeted therapy is often used for advanced kidney cancer or when the cancer has metastasized.

IMMUNOTHERAPY

This treatment boosts the body's natural defenses to fight cancer. For kidney cancer, immunotherapy may involve drugs that help the immune system recognize and destroy cancer cells more effectively. Immunotherapy has shown promising results in treating advanced or metastatic kidney cancer and is becoming an increasingly important part of treatment protocols.

SURVIVAL STATISTICS: 5-YEAR SURVIVAL RATE IS ABOUT 75%.

LIFE EXPECTANCY: Generally favorable for early-stage cancers.

PANCREATIC CANCER

CAUSES: Tobacco use significantly increases the risk of developing pancreatic cancer. Chemicals in tobacco smoke can damage the DNA of pancreatic cells, leading to cancer. Long-standing diabetes, particularly type 2, is also associated with a higher susceptibility of pancreatic cancer. The relationship is complex and may involve insulin resistance and high blood sugar levels that promote cancer growth.

Chronic inflammation of the pancreas, often due to excessive alcohol consumption or gallstones, can lead to an elevated risk of getting pancreatic cancer over time. Family history of pancreatic cancer or genetic syndromes that increase cancer risk can significantly raise an individual's risk of developing this cancer.

SYMPTOMS: Pain in the abdomen or back, often worsening at night or after eating, is a common symptom of pancreatic cancer as the tumor presses on surrounding organs or nerves. Unintentional and unexplained weight loss are also signs of many cancers, including pancreatic cancer. This may result from the body's inability to properly digest food due to the tumor blocking the pancreas.

Yellowing of the skin and eyes (Jaundice), dark urine, and light-colored stools can occur if the cancer blocks the bile duct, preventing bile from reaching the intestines and causing a buildup of bilirubin in the blood.

TREATMENTS

SURGERY

If the cancer is diagnosed early enough, surgery to remove the tumor is the most effective treatment. Procedures vary based on the tumor's location within the pancreas but may include the Whipple procedure, distal pancreatectomy, or total pancreatectomy.

CHEMOTHERAPY

Drugs that kill cancer cells are often used before surgery (neoadjuvant chemotherapy) to shrink the tumor, after surgery (adjuvant chemotherapy) to eliminate any remaining cancer cells, or as the main treatment if the cancer is inoperable.

RADIATION THERAPY

High-energy beams, such as X-rays, are used to target and kill cancer cells, often in combination with chemotherapy. Radiation therapy can help relieve symptoms and control tumor growth, especially in cases where surgery isn't possible.

SURVIVAL STATISTICS: 5-YEAR SURVIVAL RATE IS ABOUT 10%.

LIFE EXPECTANCY: Median survival is about 3 to 6 months without treatment; up to 2 years with treatment for early-stage cancer.

ESOPHAGEAL CANCER

CAUSES: The use of tobacco products significantly increases the risk of esophageal cancer. Chemicals in tobacco smoke and other products can damage the DNA of cells in the esophagus, leading to cancer.

Regular and excessive consumption of alcohol can irritate and damage the esophageal lining, increasing the risk of esophageal cancer, especially when combined with smoking.

Barrett's Esophagus, a condition often caused by chronic acid reflux (GERD), involves abnormal changes in the esophageal lining that can increase the risk of developing esophageal adenocarcinoma (cancer).

Excess body weight can lead to increased pressure on the stomach and frequent acid reflux, which may damage the lining of the esophagus over time and increase cancer risk.

SYMPTOMS: One of the earliest signs of esophageal cancer is a sensation that food is getting stuck in your throat or chest, or even pain when swallowing, as the tumor grows and narrows the esophagus.

Pain or discomfort in the chest, not necessarily related to eating, can also be a symptom of esophageal cancer.

Unintentional weight loss without trying can occur because swallowing difficulties lead to eating less and a general decrease in nutrient absorption.

TREATMENTS

SURGERY

For localized esophageal cancer, surgery to remove the affected section of the esophagus and nearby lymph nodes is a common treatment. The remaining esophagus is then reconnected to the stomach.

CHEMOTHERAPY

Cancer-fighting drugs may be used before surgery to shrink the tumor or after surgery to kill any remaining cancer cells. Chemotherapy is also an option for advanced esophageal cancer to help relieve symptoms and extend life.

RADIATION THERAPY

High-energy beams, such as X-rays, are used to target and kill cancer cells. Radiation therapy is often combined with chemotherapy (chemoradiation) and may be used before surgery to shrink the tumor or as a palliative treatment to relieve symptoms in advanced cases.

SURVIVAL STATISTICS: 5-year survival rate is about 20%.

LIFE EXPECTANCY: Varies based on stage; generally lower for advanced stages.

STOMACH (GASTRIC) CANCER

CAUSES: Helicobacter pylori infection is a common bacterial infection that causes ulcers and inflammation in the stomach lining and is a significant risk factor for developing stomach cancer.

A diet high in smoked, salted, or pickled foods can increase the risk of stomach cancer, possibly due to the carcinogenic compounds formed during the preservation process.

Having close relatives who have been diagnosed with stomach cancer increases an individual's risk, pointing towards a genetic predisposition to the disease.

SYMPTOMS: Discomfort or pain in the stomach area, which may be persistent or intermittent, is a common symptom of stomach cancer as is unintended weight loss, not associated with dieting or exercise.

Frequent nausea or vomiting, especially after meals, can indicate stomach cancer, especially if these symptoms persist over time.

TREATMENTS

SURGERY

The primary treatment for localized stomach cancer, involving the removal of the cancerous part of the stomach and sometimes nearby lymph nodes. For more advanced cases, surgery may help relieve symptoms.

CHEMOTHERAPY

Uses drugs to kill cancer cells, often given before surgery (neoadjuvant chemotherapy) to shrink the tumor or after surgery (adjuvant chemotherapy) to eliminate any remaining cancer cells. It's also used as a standalone treatment for advanced stomach cancer.

RADIATION THERAPY

This treatment uses high-energy rays to target and kill cancer cells. It may be used alongside chemotherapy before or after surgery or as a palliative treatment to relieve symptoms in advanced cases.

TARGETED THERAPY

These drugs target specific genes, proteins, or the tissue environment that contributes to cancer growth and survival. Targeted therapy is an option for certain types of stomach cancer, often based on the tumor's genetic makeup

SURVIVAL STATISTICS: 5-YEAR SURVIVAL RATE IS ABOUT 32%.

LIFE EXPECTANCY: Varies; early detection improves outcomes.

Please note: All of the survival and life expectancy rates on this page are generalized and can vary based on numerous factors, including the stage at diagnosis, overall health, response to treatment, and advancements in medical technology. Early detection and treatment are key to improving outcomes in most types of cancer.

NOT ALL CANCERS ARE EQUAL

It's important to keep in mind that certain types of cancer are inherently less aggressive. An example of this is basal cell carcinoma (BCC) which is the most common form of skin cancer. It accounts for about 80% of all skin cancers. The occurrence of basal cell carcinoma has been increasing over the years, largely due to such factors as overexposure to ultraviolet (UV) radiation from the sun and tanning beds, increased cancer screenings and an aging of the world's population.

In the United States, millions of cases of basal cell carcinoma are diagnosed each year. While it is more common in individuals with fair skin, it can occur in people of all skin types.

Basal cell carcinoma typically develops on areas of the skin that are more frequently exposed to the sun, such as the face, ears, neck, scalp, shoulders, and back. This is a type of cancer known for its slow growth and rarity in spreading to other body parts.

Similarly, some prostate cancers grow very slowly and typically don't cause significant harm over a person's lifetime.

The growth or malignancy of cancer depends greatly on its type and in its various stages. Early-stage cancers, like stage I lung cancer, the disease is relatively small and confined to the lungs. In this stage, the tumor is typically no larger than 4 cm in diameter and has not spread to any lymph nodes or distant organs. Stage I cancers are usually less aggressive and have higher survival rates compared to advanced stages like stage IV, which indicates spreading.

A cancer's growth rate plays a crucial role in how it impacts the body. Some cancers grow so slowly that they might not cause serious harm for many years, especially in elderly patients who might even outlive these cancers.

Also, response to cancer treatment varies; certain cancers, including some leukemias and lymphomas, respond well to treatments and can often be put into long-term remission, despite their potential aggressiveness.

Indolent cancers, which progress very slowly and cause minimal or no symptoms, might not necessitate immediate treatment. These cancers are often managed through "active surveillance."

In certain cases, hormone sensitivity allows cancers to be effectively controlled with hormone therapies which reduces their aggressiveness and spread.

Genetic factors significantly influence the aggressiveness of cancer. Advances in genetics have shown that specific mutations can be targeted by therapies to control or slow down the disease's progression.

CANCER AND QUALITY OF LIFE

Treatability and survivability of the most commons forms of cancer depend on several crucial factors, including what type of cancer is diagnosed, at which stage it was confirmed, the overall health of the patient and availability of effective treatments.

Even if you are diagnosed with a non-aggressive type of cancer, that's not to say that a diagnosis won't come with a tumultuous reaction emotionally, or, that it won't impact our quality of life profoundly.

While not all cancers can be entirely eradicated, most treatment strategies, including pain management, will try to minimize discomfort and add quality to life. Depending of course on how early the cancer was discovered, today's treatments stand a good chance at extending life as well.

Treatment decisions for non-aggressive cancers aim to balance the benefits of treatment against potential side effects. In some cases, aggressive treatments might not significantly extend life and could diminish the quality of life.

It's important to keep in mind here that individual risk factors for getting cancer can be influenced by lifestyle choices and or genetic predispositions.

Some cancers, like thyroid, testicular, and prostate cancer, when detected early, generally have high survival rates. Others, including pancreatic and lung cancer, are often diagnosed at both a later stage of the disease and in patients that are older and less resilient to aggressive treatment. Subsequently, survival rates are often lower for these types of cancers.

STAGE OF DIAGNOSIS

Early detection is key for successful treatment. Cancers detected at an early stage, before they have spread (metastasized), are generally more treatable and have a considerably higher survival rate. For instance, early-stage, skin melanoma, and colorectal cancers (colon) have relatively high survival rates.

ADVANCES IN TREATMENT

The development of new and more effective treatments, such as targeted therapies, immunotherapies, and precision medicine, has improved the prospect for many cancer patients. These treatments also have fewer side effects and are often more effective than traditional therapies like chemotherapy and radiation.

OVERALL HEALTH AND MULTIPLE DIAGNOSIS

Our overall health, age, and the presence of other medical conditions can affect the outcome of cancer treatment. The healthier we are at the onset, the more likely it is that we'll tolerate aggressive treatments and subsequently improve our ability to survive.

ACCESS TO HEALTHCARE

Early screening, accurate diagnosis, and effective treatments significantly influence cancer survival rates. Sadly, there is still a notable disparity in cancer outcomes between developed and developing countries, and even within countries, due to differences in financial situations and healthcare access.

LIFESTYLE FACTORS

Post-diagnosis, lifestyle factors such as diet, physical activity, and avoiding tobacco and excessive alcohol can play a significant role in treatment success and overall prognosis.

THE GOOD NEWS

The brutal truth is that if you live long enough, you will likely be diagnosed with some form of cancer.

But the good news is that since research and the development of cancer science is far from stagnant, the longer you do live, the more likely it is that there will be a treatment developed for the type of cancer you've might be diagnosed with.

The fact is that the iteration pace and evolution of cancer research is expected to increase exponentially, in no small way thanks to extensive research within artificial intelligence and quantum computing.

Using AI, genetic, clinical, and lifestyle data can be analysed with greater accuracy allowing the development of more personalized treatment strategies. And by understanding a patient's unique cancer profile, *artificial intelligence* can recommend the most effective treatments with the least side effects, tailored specifically to the individual.

In the future, Quantum computing's unique ability to analyze extremely large datasets is expected to be leveraged in oncology for pattern recognition, identifying trends in cancer progression, predicting cancer susceptibility and detecting cancer from medical images with higher accuracy.

By analyzing, simulating and predicting the interaction between different drug molecules and specific cancer proteins can potentially reduce both the development time and costs associated with new cancer treatments.

CHAPTER 7

The Aging Man's Survival Guide

YOUR PROSTATE

What it does and why it can become an issue.

This chapter is designed to explain the functions and significance of the prostate gland, alongside my own personal experiences with prostate issues that I've had to deal with. I've also included practical advice.

You'll learn about the prostate's role in the male reproductive system, explore common prostate issues including prostatitis, and discover various methods and techniques for assessing your prostate's health. I've included insights on how dietary choices and exercise can alleviate both temporary and chronic pain and discomfort associated with prostate problems.

THE PROSTATE

The prostate is a little walnut-shaped gland nestled within the male reproductive system. It's located below the bladder and in front of the rectum and though your prostate might not be very big or well-known among us men, it still plays a crucial role in our lives.

SEMEN

Seminal fluid, also known as semen, is produced in several different parts of the male reproductive system. The composition of semen is meticulously designed to optimize the survival and function of sperm within the female reproductive tract.

This complex fluid contains a mixture of substances, including spermatozoa, fructose for energy, enzymes, and various other proteins and minerals that create a protective and nourishing environment.

These components collaborate to neutralize the acidic environment of the vagina, create a conducive medium for sperm mobility, and support the sperm's journey through the cervix, into the uterus, and ultimately to the fallopian tubes where fertilization happens.

The composition of these fluids is crucial as it helps to preserve the sperm and provide the necessary energy for their long journey, thereby enhancing the likelihood of successful fertilization of the egg.

SEMEN PRODUCTION

Seminal Vesicles: About 60-70% of the semen volume is produced by the seminal vesicles, small glands located behind the bladder and above the prostate gland. This fluid is rich in fructose, which provides energy for the sperm.

Bulbourethral Glands (Cowper's Glands). These are pea-sized glands located below the prostate gland, at the base of the penis, right below the prostate and adjacent to the urethra.

These glands contribute a smaller amount of fluid compared to the seminal vesicles and prostate. They produce a clear, slippery fluid that is released before ejaculation to help lubricate the urethra for sperm to pass through more easily and neutralize any traces of acidic urine in the urethra.

Prostate Gland: The prostate contributes approximately 30% of the seminal fluid in semen. This fluid contains enzymes like PSA (prostate-specific antigen), as well as other substances that help sperm function more effectively and survive longer. This seminal fluid is a key component of semen, the medium through which sperm are transported during ejaculation.

The prostate's secretion serves multiple crucial functions: it helps to maintain the optimal concentration of sperm by contributing to the volume of semen, facilitates ejaculation, and provides essential nutrients and enzymes. These nutrients and enzymes support sperm viability and promote motility, which are important for successful fertilization.

THROUGH YOUR URETHRA

The prostate strategically wraps around the beginning of the urethra – the channel for both urine and semen. While urine is normally the main fluid, during ejaculation, the prostate ensures that only the finest batch of semen gets the green light to race up the urethra, the inside your penis.

HORMONE PRODUCTION

The prostate also plays a part in maintaining hormonal balance, particularly the male sex hormones, like testosterone. The reduction in testosterone levels can lead to symptoms commonly associated with male aging, including decreased muscle and bone mass, reduced sexual function and drive, fatigue, and mood swings.

The interplay between prostate health and hormone regulation underscores the importance of the prostate gland in overall male well-being, especially during the later stages of life.

PROSTATITIS

Despite its important contributing status, your prostate isn't immune to causing problems. Which seems like a perfect segue to talk about the dreaded – but treatable – inflammation of the prostate, so-called Prostatitis.

Prostatitis is the medical term used to describe inflammation of the prostate gland. It can have various causes, and affect men of all ages in many different ways. For men aged 55 and older, prostatitis can manifest through a variety of symptoms, making it a condition that can significantly impact your quality of life.

Commonly symptoms include a persistent urge to urinate, difficulty starting urination or a weak urine stream, vague discomfort or pain in the pelvic area, mild aching in the lower back, or genital area, and even a painful ejaculation.

Flu-like symptoms may also arise, particularly in cases of acute bacterial prostatitis. Frequent nighttime urination and discomfort or burning sensation during urination are typical, underscoring the discomfort and disruption Prostatitis can cause to daily activities and sleep.

If you have one or several of these symptoms, it's important that you see a healthcare professional, preferably a urologist, as soon as possible to have your prostate examined.

WHAT TO EXPECT DURING YOUR FIRST VISIT TO A UROLOGIST

First a little of my personal experiences that you will hopefully find helpful (but that might also cause a little anxiety, read on with caution).

Over the years, I've probably seen at least three dozen doctors specialized in urology as well as general practitioners that seemed knowledgable enough to perform a prostate examination with some confidence.

Back in the early 1980s, when I had just turned 20, for whatever underlying reason (which to this day is unbeknownst to me), I started experiencing issues with my prostate. At the time, I didn't even know what a prostate was, much less why I had one.

So I was completely ignorant that this thing called a prostate could succumb to an inflammation or how mine got inflamed.

Despite several examinations and treatments with wide-spectrum antibiotics (and insertions of anti-inflammatory suppositories), the pain from my stubborn prostate persisted. Eventually, after about a year of consistently failing treatments, I was diagnosed with Prostatitis.

This chronic condition lasted for a couple of years during which I probably had my prostate examined via my anus a dozen times at multiple clinics by as many prostate probing Urologists.

(When I think about those days of prostate woes, it occurs to me that I certainly had a lot of fingers rummaging around in my behind).

As the antibiotic treatment prescribed by the various urologists I saw didn't do much to ease my inflammation or discomfort, one of them finally suggested that I undergo a so-called cystoscopy – a procedure that involves inserting a lensed tube deep into the penis to allow a doctor to examine my bladder and urethra, the narrow yet elastic pathway that carries urine and semen out of the male body.

I can't emphasize enough how painful this procedure was and how terrible I felt afterwards. Now, at the time, I might have had a ridiculously low pain threshold. But before my second cystoscopy examination, yes, I had not one but two, I insisted on full anesthesia and my Urologist at the time obliged my request.

While being under anesthesia meant that I didn't have to endure the pain from the actual insertion and probing process of the cystoscope, for several hours afterwards, I still ended up walking bent over at a 70 degree angle.

And the first few times I urinated after the cystoscope rod had been pulled out of my penis, it felt like an endless river of molten lava was slowly flowing and dripping from my penis.

Eventually, about two years after my prostate ordeal had begun, the prostatitis subsided and all symptoms vanished as mysteriously as they had appeared.

WHAT TO EXPECT: YOUR FIRST UROLOGICAL EXAMINATION

A urological examination for a man over 50 typically focuses on assessing the health of your urinary and reproductive system, as well as screening for common conditions that become more prevalent as we age. Here are some of the topics you can expect to be discussed and inspected during your first visit with a Urologist

MEDICAL HISTORY

The urologist will likely begin by asking you about your medical history, including any existing medical conditions, medications, surgeries, and family history of urological issues.

PHYSICAL EXAMINATION

You can also expect some degree of physical examination that includes checking your vital signs, examining the abdomen, groin, and genital area for any abnormalities or signs of inflammation.

DIGITAL RECTAL EXAM (DRE)

This is the typical part of a urological exam for aging men. We'll dig deeper into this topic in a bit.

URINALYSIS

You may be asked for a urine sample to analyze for signs of urinary tract infections, blood in the urine, or other abnormalities.

PROSTATE-SPECIFIC ANTIGEN (PSA) TEST

This common blood test measures the level of PSA, a protein produced by your prostate gland. Elevated PSA levels can indicate prostate issues, including prostate cancer. It's worth noting that interpretation and implications can vary with PSA testing and could be followed by your Urologist's decision to proceed with further testing or treatment if deemed necessary.

ULTRASOUND

Depending on the findings from the physical exam and PSA test, the doctor might recommend a transrectal ultrasound to get a clearer view of the prostate gland and surrounding structures. More about this in a while.

UROFLOWMETRY

This test measures the rate of urine flow during urination. It can help identify problems with urine flow due to an enlarged prostate or other urinary issues.

CYSTOSCOPY

In some cases, a flexible or rigid cystoscope – a thin tube with a camera on the end – might be inserted through your penis to visualize the bladder and urethra. This can help identify issues such as bladder stones, tumors, or urethral strictures. We'll also cover more of this procedure further on.

BONE DENSITY TEST

Osteoporosis, a condition characterized by weakened bones, becomes more common with age. Depending on your risk factors, a bone density test might be recommended to assess your bone health.

DISCUSSION AND RECOMMENDATIONS

Based on findings and test results, your Urologist will want to discuss your urological health, provide any necessary recommendations for treatment or further evaluation, and address any concerns or questions you might have.

WHY WE GET PROSTATITIS

BACTERIAL INFECTION

Prostatitis can be caused by a bacterial infection. Bacteria from the

*urinary tract or elsewhere in the body can find its way into the pros-
tate, and lead to inflammation. This is known as bacterial prostatitis
and can be either acute or chronic. I've had both and sincerely hope
you experience neither.*

NON-BACTERIAL INFLAMMATION

Sometimes prostatitis occurs without a bacterial infection. This
somewhat mystical cause is called non-bacterial prostatitis or
chronic pelvic pain syndrome (CPPS).

URINARY TRACT INFECTIONS (UTIS)

Infections in the urinary tract, including the bladder and urethra,
can sometimes spread to the prostate, leading to prostatitis.

SEXUALLY TRANSMITTED INFECTIONS (STIS)

If left untreated for too long, sexually transmitted infections, such
as gonorrhea or chlamydia, can cause prostatitis.

URINARY RETENTION

Incomplete emptying of the bladder can lead to stagnant urine, creating an environment where bacteria can multiply and cause prostatitis. While you might not want to spoil your bladder with too frequent pees, according to urologists I've spoken to, emptying your
bladder completely each time you do pee is important.

TRAUMA

Physical trauma or injury to the perineum – the area between your
scrotum (ballsack) and your anus – can lead to inflammation in the
prostate and worse yet, prostatitis.

URINARY CATHETERIZATION

If you're unlucky, using a non-sterile urinary catheter can introduce
bacteria into the urinary tract and prostate, increasing the risk of
infection and kickstarting an inflammation.

IMMUNE SYSTEM FACTORS

Some men may be more susceptible to prostatitis due to underlying immune system issues caused by illness or immune suppressant
medication.

Ok, so now lets dig into the various prostate examination methods.

DRE

The most common type of prostate inspection is a so-called Digital Rectal Examination (DRE). Here, digital means finger, as in a Urologists index finger, which is exactly what he or she is going to use to assess the size, shape, and texture of your prostate through your anal cavity.

PREPARATION

There are no outspoken requirements to go on a fast prior to a DRE, but if possible, I strongly suggest you try to have a thorough bowel movement before your prostate examination. This will make the procedure less uncomfortable for both you and the Urologist who will be poking through your anus in order to reach up until he locates your prostate gland.

Once you arrive at the Urologist's clinic or a hospital, and perhaps after a brief discussion about your condition and medical history or any specific concerns you may have, the doctor will unceremoniously ask you to either change into a gown or just lower your pants and underwear down to your shoes.

You'll most likely be asked to position yourself either lying on your side with your knees drawn up to your chest or bending over the examination table. I've personally never experienced having to bend over a examination table, but I still wanted to at least mention it as a possible alternative.

GLOVES AND LUBRICATION

While you are getting ready for the examination, the Urologist will be gloving up and then applying a generous amount of lubricant to his or her index finger. This is done to ensure a smooth anal insertion and frictionless probing of your prostate.

INSERTION

With the gloved and lubricated finger, your Urologist will then gently (hopefully) insert his finger into your rectum. We all experience this differently, somewhat depending on sexual preference and the thickness of the doctor's finger, but most men would agree that this feels slightly weird and uncomfortable, yet not terribly painful. Don't hesitate to let your Urologist know if you have any significant discomfort.

FEELING THE PROSTATE

Once the Urologist's finger is deep enough inside your body, they will locate and then with their finger feel the surface of your prostate gland, its size, shape, texture, and any unusual lumps or abnormalities it may have. This part of the examination is relatively quick and typically lasts 15-30 seconds.

FEEDBACK

After the examination, your Urologist will discuss their findings with you. They may convey whether the prostate feels normal or if there are any concerns that require further investigation, such as a biopsy or additional imaging.

TRANSRECTAL ULTRASOUND EXAMINATION (TRUS)

If your urologist determines that further evaluation of the prostate is needed, they may suggest a transrectal ultrasound (TRUS), which provides a more detailed view of the gland.

HOW A TRUS IS PERFORMED

PREPARATION

You may need to drink water and refrain from eating for several hours before this procedure. With your bowel empty, it will be easier to capture a clear image of the prostate. As with the DRE, you'll likely be asked to change into a gown or pull down your pants and underwear before the examination begins.

POSITIONING

You'll be positioned similarly to the DRE, either on your side or possibly bending over the examination table.

THE PROBE

Here's when a small device, an ultrasound probe which is about the size of a thick middle finger that has hopefully been generously coated with a transparent or semi-transparent gel is inserted into your anus.

The probe emits high-frequency sound waves, which when bounced back and sent to a screen, create real-time images of your prostate.

IMAGE CAPTURE

The urologist will slowly move the ultrasound probe within the rectum to capture images of the surrounding areas of the prostate. This inspection can take longer (than a DRE) and you may well feel more pressure and an increase in discomfort than during the Digital Rectal Examination, but it's generally not too painful unless you have hemorrhoids or other intestinal issues.

EVALUATION

After the images are obtained through the ultrasound probe, your Urologist will carefully examines the images to ascertain the prostate's size, shape, and any potential abnormalities, such as tumors or enlarged areas.

DISCUSSION

Once this examination is complete, your Urologist will discuss the findings with you. They may recommend further tests or procedures based on the ultrasound results. Or, hopefully, send you on your merry way with the scientific knowledge that your prostate gland is in good shape.

PSA SCREENING

A Prostate-Specific Antigen (PSA) test is a blood test primarily used to screen for prostate cancer. The test measures the level of PSA, a protein produced by both cancerous and noncancerous tissue in the prostate, a small gland that sits below the bladder in men. PSA is present in small quantities in the blood of healthy men, but elevated levels can indicate prostate cancer, benign prostate enlargement (BPH), inflammation of the prostate (prostatitis), or other conditions.

The PSA test result is usually reported as nanograms of PSA per milliliter (ng/mL) of blood. Reading the results:

0 to 2.5 ng/mL is considered a low PSA level, suggesting a low risk of prostate cancer.

2.6 to 4.0 ng/mL is seen as a borderline range, and doctors may suggest a retest or further monitoring.

4.1 to 10.0 ng/mL is considered a moderately elevated range, which might indicate a higher risk of prostate cancer or other prostate conditions.

Above 10.0 ng/mL is considered high, significantly increasing the likelihood of prostate cancer.

Keep in mind that PSA levels can vary with age, and higher PSA levels are more common in older men, even without cancer. Non-cancerous conditions like BPH (Benign Prostatic Hyperplasia) can also cause elevated PSA levels.

Factors like race, family history, and certain medications can also affect PSA levels. Interpreting PSA test results isn't always straightforward and must be done by a healthcare professional who can consider all these factors.

If PSA levels are elevated, further testing, including a prostate biopsy, might be recommended to determine the cause.

Regular prostate examinations and Prostate-Specific Antigen (PSA) tests are crucial components of ensuring our health, especially as we age.

These preventative measures are recommended at least every two years as a vital way in detecting early signs of prostate issues, including prostate cancer, which can have far-reaching impacts on quality of life, relationships, and overall health.

Painful symptoms such as difficulty peeing, pelvic discomfort, or changes in urinary habits not only degrade day-to-day living but can also serve as early warning signs of more serious health issues.

Early detection through regular checkups and screenings can lead to more effective treatments, significantly improving outcomes and potentially saving your life. Given the prostate's role in hormonal balance and its impact on functions ranging from urinary flow to sexual health, maintaining vigilance through regular check-ups is an essential practice for aging men in preserving our health and well-being.

Today, almost 40 years later, some of the symptoms from that early bout of prostatitis have sadly returned and just a few months after turning 60, I was examined by a female urologist.

Fortunately, the checkup, performed first with her index finger and then a surprisingly large ultrasound probe, both adequately lubed, showed that my prostate was in reasonably good shape. My uroflowmetry test showed good urine flow and my PSA (Prostate-Specific Antigen) levels were low.

The urologist told me without much cushioning, that there was not much that could be done to help with the at times extremely frequent urination, the vague pain I often felt around my groin and other minor but noticeable symptoms caused by my aging prostate.

Before leaving her office, the urologist offered me some solid advice on how to reduce some of my discomfort and suggestions on how to maintain a healthy prostate.

Keep caffeine and alcohol consumption to a minimum.

Eat healthy food that doesn't contribute to an increase of inflammation in my body.

Do not "spoil" my bladder by urinating too often.

Exercise regularly and keep the muscles of the pelvic floor strong and elastic.

THE PELVIC FLOOR

The pelvic floor is a mesh of muscles and tissues that stretch across the base of the pelvis, supporting the bladder and bowel and contributing to sexual function.

As we men age, these muscles often get weaker or become too tight, leading to a range of issues that can include urinary incontinence, difficulties with bowel control, erectile dysfunction, and a numbness or abstract pain in the pelvic area.

Regular exercises aimed at strengthening the pelvic floor, can help mitigate these issues and improve quality of life as we get older.

Here are some exercises that may help you alleviate discomfort that can be caused by the prostate.

KEGEL EXERCISES

These exercises for strengthening the pelvic floor muscles, which support bladder, bowel and urinary control.

To perform Kegels, tighten the muscles you would use to stop urinating midstream, hold for 3-5 seconds, and then relax for 3-5 seconds. Repeat this 10-15 times per session, aiming for at least three sessions a day.

PELVIC FLOOR "LIFTS"

Similar to Kegels but with a focus on "lifting" the pelvic floor upwards. Imagine lifting the entire pelvic floor towards your belly button. Hold the lift for a few seconds and then release gently.

Please note: Getting guidance from a physical therapist or healthcare provider will ensure that you have the correct technique and effectiveness for both Kegel and Pelvic Floor exercises.

BRIDGE POSE

Lie on your back with knees bent and feet flat on the ground, hip-width apart. Press your feet into the ground and lift your hips towards the ceiling, squeezing the buttocks at the top.

This move strengthens the lower back and pelvic floor muscles. Hold for a few seconds before slowly lowering the hips back down.

PILATES

While primarily focusing on core strength, pilates also engages and strengthens the pelvic floor muscles. Exercises like the Pilates bridge, leg lifts, and pelvic tilts can be particularly helpful.

YOGA

Certain yoga poses can help stretch and strengthen the pelvic floor muscles, reduce stress, and improve circulation.

Poses like Child's Pose, Reclining Bound Angle Pose, and Gentle Seated Twist can offer relief.

WALKING

Regular, gentle walking can help reduce stress, improve circulation, and maintain overall pelvic health without putting too much strain on the body.

AEROBIC EXERCISES

Low-impact aerobic exercises, like swimming or cycling, can improve blood flow and help reduce symptoms associated with prostate pain.

Understanding the functions of the prostate, potential issues like prostatitis, and the methods for maintaining prostate health are not just academic exercises – they are vital, actionable steps that can significantly enhance your quality of life if and when you have issues related to your prostate.

Knowledge is power, especially when it comes to health. By staying informed about the signs and symptoms of prostate problems, you are now hopefully better prepared to act swiftly. Coupled with regular screenings and medical check-ups, this should empower you to catch potential problems early, when they are most treatable.

CHAPTER 8

The Aging Man's Survival Guide

NAVIGATING CHANGE: AGING & SEXUALITY

Benefits of keeping your sex drive alive and prostate healthy.

In this chapter, we'll explore the physical changes the male sexual organs go through with aging, including functionality and shifts in size. You'll also read about how our libido, or sex drive, can be impacted and the psychological implications this can have and the importance of accepting these changes as a natural part of life.

THE EBB AND FLOW OF SEXUAL DESIRE

From the enthusiastic curiosity and intense sex drive of our younger days to the more relaxed rhythm of later years, the way we express our sexuality evolves as we age. Each overlapping era comes with its own challenges and joys, each adding valuable experiences to the ongoing story of our sex life.

Young Adulthood (Teens to 20s)

This is typically a time of curiosity and discovery, where sexual desire and the frequency of ejaculation and orgasms are often at their peak. It's a period of learning, experimentation, and, for many, the most active phase of sexual exploration.

ADULTHOOD (30S TO 50S)

Life's responsibilities may begin to interfere with the frequency of sexual activity, but for many, it remains a big part of life. This is also a time for deepening intimacy, exploring desires, and for some, starting families.

MIDDLE AGE (50S AND BEYOND)

Changes in sexual function can become more pronounced in this period, with fluctuations in sexual activity, sex drive, and for some men, a disruption in erectile function. This can also be a time of sexual renaissance, discovering new sources of pleasure and intimacy.

OLDER AGE (70S AND BEYOND)

While frequency may decrease, the capacity for pleasure and intimacy can be unchanged and even increase. For some, this phase can represent a shift towards the qualitative aspects of sex, focusing more on intimacy, touch, and connection.

UNDERSTANDING AND EMBRACING CHANGE

Our sexual drive and the frequency of when we have sex changes as we grow older. Recognizing, accepting, and adapting to these natural changes can help us create a deeper appreciation of our sexual needs and desires – regardless of age.

In the last five years, since turning 55, my relationship with intimacy has undergone a series of changes physically and emotionally. After initially grappling with the changes, the transformation has since brought a more relaxed attitude towards sex.

While it's undeniable that my desire for sex has decreased with age, I've come to the insight that this is actually okay and that non-sexual intimacy can sometimes even transcend the act of sex.

There's a common misconception that sexual desire diminishes entirely as we age. Though true that hormonal changes and physical limitations might contribute to a decline in our sex drive, the need for intimacy can instead increase as we get older.

In younger years, my wife and I frequently enjoyed spontaneous sex. The frequency and intensity of our lovemaking seemed insatiable and we made love anywhere at any time of day or night.

As we've aged, and especially after menopause, there's been a noticeable decrease in my wife's need to have sex. She still enjoys herself when we are sexually intimate, but it's not nearly as often as when we were younger.

According to recent research, *statistically, men think about sex roughly twice as often as women do, 19 vs 10 times per day.*

At first, I struggled with feelings of nostalgia for those years of vigorous, passionate sex with my wife. I've even sometimes wondered if a decrease in our sex life would also signal a decline in our relationship.

I've since come to realize that physical intimacy is not solely defined by sex. It's found in the tender moments of affectionate gestures, the shared laughter over our inside jokes, and the companionship of watching a movie together.

Closeness encompasses a wider spectrum of emotional, psychological, and physical connections that have helped deepen and strengthen our relationship.

Communication played a pivotal role in how we navigated this transition. An open and honest dialogue allowed us to express our desires and insecurities without judging each other and we soon realized that our bond transcended physicality; it was rooted in mutual respect, trust and in our long friendship.

As we embrace intimacy in later life, it's important to dispel societal myths and expectations surrounding men's aging and sexuality.

Contrary to popular belief, desire and pleasure are not confined to youth; they are enduring facets of the human experience that evolve over time. By redefining our understanding of intimacy, we can also cultivate fulfilling and meaningful relationships well into our later years.

By prioritizing communication, mutual respect, and shared experiences, my wife and I have discovered a profound sense of fulfillment and joy in our relationship. Ultimately, intimacy is not bound by age or libido; it's a journey of love that evolves throughout our lives.

I think it's essential to understand and accept the role of physical health in shaping our experiences of intimacy as we age. While aging may bring with it certain limitations, maintaining good overall health through regular exercise and eating well can have a really positive impact on our sexual desire, our vitality and our attractiveness.

Also, asking for guidance from healthcare professionals can help us with underlying issues that may affect sexual function and sex drive.

MALE SEX DRIVE

Whether you agree or not, some theories in evolutionary psychology suggest that men are biologically "programmed" to seek multiple partners to increase their chances of reproductive success.

This theory is partly based on that historically, men tend to have shorter lifespans due to higher rates of risk-taking and propensity to be involved in violence. As a result, it's argued that men have evolved to have a stronger sex drive to maximize their reproductive opportunities within a potentially shorter lifespan.

From a young age, boys often receive both social and cultural signals about what it means to be a "real man," which typically includes being sexually proactive and controlling. This kind of social conditioning can influence our social behavior – as well as self-perception – even if it doesn't align with our individual preferences.

As we age, some men, myself included, find solace in a reduced sex drive. Discovering that life can still offer profound satisfaction even without the pursuit of sex or the fulfillment it once provided is somehow liberating. Priorities shift, and other aspects of life take precedence, bringing a sense of contentment with what we have today.

This transition is entirely normal, just as it is for men who experience no discernible change in their sexual drive as they grow older and continue to enjoy a healthy sex life until their very last breath.

ERECTIONS AND MASTURBATION

For me, navigating my sexual awakening during adolescence and puberty was a whirlwind of both exciting discoveries and confusing challenges. As a teenager, I would often have unexpected, intense erections that refused to subside and could therefore become a little painful and occur in inappropriate settings, including during class. I vividly recall how I felt terribly vulnerable and unsure of how to manage this without drawing unwanted attention to the bulge in my jeans.

Learning to cope with situations like these as a young man was not just about physical discomfort or dealing with an inability to control a bodily function. They were also about mastering the art of discreetness and an internal dialogue about my masculinity.

These experiences, while certainly fraught with embarrassment, illuminated the complex interplay between the physical and psychological aspects of my sexual awakening.

Sex has always been an important part of my life. While I still believe that my frequent need for sex, on my own or together with my wife, has been within the norm, I've never seen masturbation as one of my guilty pleasures.

For me, achieving an orgasm has always been about experiencing the "release" which is how I've always been able to enjoy both immense physical pleasure and unique, post-orgasmic calmness. Oftentimes, once I am relieved, I'll usually feel less stressed and have a surge of positive energy.

In younger years, regardless of how often or with whom I had sex, the frequency of pleasuring myself was not necessarily impacted. Having an orgasm 5-7 times per week, in addition to having sex with my partner, wasn't at all unusual.

Some might argue that this frequency could be classified as an addiction. Yet, statistically, the ratio is not regarded as abnormal. Sex addiction is a real problem for many men – and some women – and I believe that online pornography has certainly exacerbated it. Worse yet, some porn has indirectly legitimized extreme sexual violence and introduced and/or augmented fantasies that portray and glamorize nonconsensual sex.

Admittedly, there have been periods in my life when I wished there wasn't as much pornography so easily accessible online.

ORGASM VS EJACULATION

As we grow older, how we experience the climactic phase of sex can also change, so I think it's appropriate to insert the distinctions between ejaculation and orgasm here.

EJACULATION

Physically, an ejaculation is primarily a reflex action controlled by the autonomic nervous system and happens when semen is expelled from the body through the penis. This is a physical response that involves the contraction of muscles around the base of the penis, prostate gland, and other areas of the reproductive system, pushing the semen out.

ORGASM

Neurologically, an orgasm involves the release of chemicals in the brain, including endorphins and oxytocin, which can induce feelings of euphoria and relaxation. Orgasms can happen with or without the process of ejaculation and are experienced very differently. This is the peak of sexual pleasure, characterized by intense sensations of pleasure and accompanied by a series of rhythmic contractions in the pelvic region.

SHAPE SHIFTING

Unsurprisingly, your penis is as unique as you are. And like it or not, just as with you, over the years, some remarkable changes in its guise and functionality will inevitably begin to appear.

If you're anything like me, at times over-aware, hyper-sensitive and periodically paranoid, I strongly urge you to read on and both confront and own these changes.

I've found that by at least trying to deal with unavoidable "modifications" of my physicality with a reasonable level of fatalism, a dash of humor and on occasion a straightforward dialogue with my wife, I've found that accepting them is a whole lot easier.

I'm not providing any guidelines or guarantees whatsoever, but by opening up about this unpreventable change, the journey could become less daunting and maybe, even a bit interesting.

As we age, our penis experiences a series of quite noticeable cosmetic and physiological (functional) changes. These changes can affect us in profound ways, so it is important to keep in mind that you're not alone. In one way or another, this happens to us all.

SIZE AND APPEARANCE

Just as wrinkles inevitably appear on our faces with age, your penis will also undergo some cosmetic changes. Due to the reduced blood flow and less tissue elasticity, your penis will eventually become smaller. And because the skin surrounding it is going to get thinner and less tight, the texture will eventually remind you more of a well-worn road map than the silky smooth surface you're used to seeing, holding and feeling.

Penile shrinkage can create psychological turmoil, particularly for men who once found pride in their larger than average organs. For these individuals, the reduction isn't always merely an adjustment to the physical change in size. It can also be quite a blow to their sexual confidence and magnify anxiety around intimacy.

Conversely, men who have navigated life with what society deems a 'normal' or a smaller than normal penis, might find the transition less jarring, having already embraced a sense of sexual competence that isn't tethered to size alone.

This highlights a crucial perspective: that the ability to pleasure a partner or conceive life usually transcends the physical appearance and dimensions of a man's penis.

Again, even a significant reduction in size, while emotionally challenging for some, does not detract from a man's inherent capacity to experience and provide sexual pleasure or to fulfill the biological imperative of procreation.

The scrotum or ballsack, may also lose some of its elasticity, causing it to hang lower than in younger years. This phenomenon, informally known as "switch," occurs when the scrotum extends below the length of the tip of the penis.

While these changes are typically a natural part of aging, they can also impact a man's self-esteem and body image. It's important to understand that these changes are very common and that discussing them openly can provide some reassurance that these changes are a natural part of aging and something most men experience.

HEALTH AND ORGASM

Some men over 60, myself included, experience the sensation from an orgasm to be stronger than before. It isn't always as lengthy as it once was, but the light that burns twice as bright shines half as long…

Pleasure aside, perhaps the most important reason to continue having regular orgasms, especially for aging men, is the fact that frequent ejaculation has been proven to reduce the risk of prostate cancer.

Men that ejaculate multiple times a week are much less likely to get prostate cancer before the age of 70 than men who ejaculated less frequently.

Of course, we are all different and so our individual sexual interests and preferences will vary, particularly as we get older. But I still want to share an overview of some of the physical and mental benefits of the male orgasm and ejaculation, how frequency and volume of semen may change as we age, and how all this is in fact a natural part of male aging.

Orgasms, which most men see as the ultimate goal of sexual activity, have several positive effects on both the body and mind.

PAIN RELIEF

The path to orgasm is not merely a pursuit of pleasure but can also be a significant pain relieving experience. The release of endorphins during an orgasm acts as a natural painkiller, offering temporary relief from various pains, from the acute discomfort of headaches to the enduring struggle against chronic pain.

This phenomenon showcases the body's incredible ability to seek comfort and healing through the realms of pleasure, emphasizing the intricate connection between pleasure and well-being.

STRESS REDUCTION

Achieving orgasm serves as a potent stress reliever, far beyond the mere physical release. The surge of endorphins, known for their stress-reducing qualities, provides a psychological reprieve, momentarily erasing the weight of daily stresses. This effect underscores the orgasm's role not just in physical satisfaction but as a sanctuary for mental health, offering a temporary retreat from the complexities of everyday life.

IMPROVED SLEEP

The tranquility that follows an orgasm paves the way for deeper and more restful sleep. This effect stems not only from a state of physical relaxation but from the profound peace that accompanies it, enhancing the quality of sleep and its restorative powers. It's a testament to how closely intertwined our sexual health is with our overall well-being.

CARDIOVASCULAR HEALTH

An orgasm does more than just elevate pleasure; it also boosts heart health by increasing heart rate and improving blood circulation. This cardiovascular workout underscores the symbiotic relationship between sexual health and heart health, highlighting the importance of pleasure in maintaining physical wellness.

IMMUNE SYSTEM BOOST

Engaging in regular sexual activities and experiencing orgasms can play a delightful role in bolstering the immune system. This intriguing interplay between sexual satisfaction and immune function suggests a joyful approach to enhancing bodily defenses, embodying the perfect union of pleasure and health.

MOOD ENHANCEMENT

The chemical cascade triggered by an orgasm acts as a natural mood enhancer, temporarily brightening one's outlook on life. This biochemical symphony orchestrated by the brain demonstrates the orgasm's power not only in providing momentary pleasure but also in offering emotional upliftment.

BONDING

The orgasmic experience, whether shared with a partner or enjoyed alone, fosters a deep sense of connection and intimacy. It's a moment of vulnerability and closeness that strengthens bonds, highlighting the profound emotional significance of this peak of pleasure.

IMPROVED SELF-ESTEEM

Experiencing orgasm can affirm one's sense of sexuality and contribute significantly to self-esteem. It serves as a powerful reminder of the body's capability for pleasure, bolstering confidence and celebrating one's sexuality as an integral part of human identity.

ENHANCING RELATIONSHIPS

The pursuit and experience of mutual pleasure through orgasms can act as a powerful adhesive in relationships, deepening emotional ties and reinforcing the bond between partners. This shared intimacy highlights the role of sexual fulfillment in nurturing a strong, enduring partnership.

BETTER BODY IMAGE

Orgasms can lead to a more positive perception of one's body by celebrating its ability to experience profound joy. This change in perspective is crucial for mental health, fostering a sense of appreciation and love for one's physical self.

For most men aged 55 and older, there's typically a noticeable decrease in the volume of semen produced, compared to the quantities generated during younger years. However, this does not imply a lack of fertility. Even with this reduction, there remains a substantial number of sperm – amounting to millions – capable of fertilizing a fertile female, should that be the goal.

DISCOLORED SEMEN

When small blood vessels in the prostate, seminal vesicles, or the ejaculatory ducts break, tiny amounts of blood can mix with semen, giving it a brownish hue. This condition, known as hematospermia, is generally benign and temporary.

The physical exertion or lower body pressure from activities like cycling can cause micro traumas. Similarly, a lack of activity can lead to congestion in the pelvic area, potentially resulting in similar outcomes.

While the sight of brown semen can be concerning, if the condition persists or is accompanied by other symptoms, seek medical consultation to rule out any serious conditions.

POST-EJACULATION DISCOMFORT

From time to time, I have experienced a low-grade pain or discomfort after ejaculation. From the urologists I've spoken with, this feeling is quite common among men 55 and older.

The cause can be attributed to various factors, and though not something to be overly concerned about, it's still wise to have a proper evaluation and diagnosis made. Especially if the pain increases over time or symptoms widen. Some potential causes of post-ejaculatory pain may include:

PROSTATITIS

Inflammation or infection of the prostate gland, known as prostatitis, can cause pain or discomfort in the pelvic area, lower abdomen, or in the area between the anus and the scrotum (perineum). Prostatitis can be acute (sudden and severe) or chronic (long-lasting), and it may lead to pain during or, after ejaculation. You can read more about *Prostatitis in the chapter* **Your Prostate**.

SEMINAL VESICULITIS

The seminal vesicles, which are glands that produce seminal fluid, can become inflamed and result in discomfort or pain in the pelvic region, especially following ejaculation.

URETHRITIS

The tube that carries urine and semen out of the body through the penis is the urethra. Inflammation in the urethra may cause pain or a burning sensation during or after ejaculation.

EPIDIDYMITIS

Inflammation or infection of the epididymis, a structure that stores and transports sperm, can lead to testicular pain or discomfort, which may be exacerbated after ejaculation.

PELVIC FLOOR DYSFUNCTION

Issues with the pelvic floor muscles can sometimes result in pain or discomfort during and after ejaculation. The pelvic floor is a group of muscles and connective tissues located at the base of the pelvis, and it plays a crucial role in supporting the organs in the pelvic region and contributes to various bodily functions.

For men, pelvic floor muscles help support and maintain the position of several important organs, including the bladder, rectum, and, the prostate gland.

The pelvic floor muscles also play an important role in urinary and bowel control. They help control the release of urine from the bladder and the passage of feces from the rectum. These muscles are also involved in achieving and maintaining erections, controlling ejaculation, and supporting sexual sensations.

Finally, the pelvic floor is essential for maintaining proper posture and stability of the pelvis and lower back.

OTHER FACTORS

Other potential causes of post-ejaculatory pain may include urinary tract infections, sexually transmitted infections, and structural abnormalities. Since the causes of post-ejaculatory pain can vary, I strongly suggest that you seek medical advice if you experience this discomfort for a prolonged period of time.

ERECTILE DYSFUNCTION

With age, the blood vessels in the penis lose their former agility, leading to slower (and not uncommonly) less stiff erections. So even though it might take longer to rise to the occasion, sometimes reaching full stiffness might take more time.

Here is where foreplay can make a game-changing difference for men. And with foreplay, I include anything that could help with a slightly or fully dysfunctional erection, including – but not limited to – the four most popular so-called PDE5 inhibitors also known as erectile enhancing medications, like Avanafil (Stendra), Sildenafil (Viagra), Tadalafil (Cialis) and Vardenafil.

Some find viewing pornography, using sex toys and applying lubricants can help getting an uncooperative penis into one ready for ejaculation and orgasm, including oral, vaginal or anal penetration.

Keep in mind that with age, some men experience both premature and delayed ejaculation, which can possibly lead to frustrating experiences for both you and your partner.

OVERALL HEALTH IMPACT

The penis, being a part of the whole of you, is affected by your overall health. Lifestyle choices, including diet, fitness, and, of course, intake of alcohol, recreational drugs and smoking can influence your ability to enjoy sex as you age.

Your brain will also play a pivotal role in how your sex life evolves as you get older. Stress, anxiety, and psychological factors can impact performance and enjoyment.

At 60, I feel that this topic should be ridden with less fraught with drama and stigma. Sadly, just as with our health, it's something we men talk very little about, especially with each other. At least on a serious level. More on this in the chapter **Health Secrecy**.

Hopefully, this is not the case when it comes to your significant other. I've always found that having an open dialogue about even the most sensitive topics is always preferable to keeping them closed off.

PROSTATE HEALTH

As discussed in the previous chapter, "Your Prostate," the prostate gland plays an important role in male reproductive health by producing a significant portion of the fluid that comprises semen. This fluid not only nourishes and helps transport sperm, it also protects individual sperm and enhances motility, which is crucial for their fertility.

Encouraging the prostate to fully empty its contents can be beneficial for several reasons. First, it makes sure that the gland is functioning optimally.

Regular ejaculation, whether through sex or prostate stimulation, helps to clear the ducts within the prostate, which in turn reduces the buildup of old fluid and potential irritants. This process may lower the risk of prostatic congestion and inflammation, conditions that can lead to both a general sense of discomfort and chronic prostate issues, including prostatitis.

Regularly emptying the prostate can contribute to improved overall prostate function by maintaining the elasticity of the prostate tissue. This is particularly important as we age and the risk of benign prostatic hyperplasia (BPH) and other prostate-related issues increases.

There is also evidence to suggest that frequent ejaculation may have a protective effect against prostate cancer. Some studies have indicated that regular ejaculation results in a lower concentration of cancer-causing substances in the prostate gland, thereby potentially reducing the risk of developing cancer.

EMPTYING THE PROSTATE GLAND

With some practice, the prostate gland can easily be emptied by becoming more mindful about the final climactic phase that precedes ejaculation.

By relaxing your abdominal, groin and entire pelvic area several seconds prior to the "point of no return" has been reached, when ejaculation and orgasm are just moments away, the prostate gland is provided with a better opportunity to completely empty its seminal fluid.

For many men, this method can also enhance sexual pleasure, as the technique extends the duration and intensity of the climatic experience. By simply focusing on the process and increasing awareness of our body's responses, we not only support physical health but we can also elevate our sexual wellbeing.

PROSTATE MILKING

The term "prostate milking" is a therapeutic prostate massage that is used to reduce symptoms related to various prostate conditions. Prostate Milking can be performed by healthcare professionals or with guidance at home and involves specific techniques designed to gently stimulate the prostate gland.

Prostate milking is designed to stimulate blood flow and fluid secretion. The pressure applied should be firm but not painful. Techniques can vary depending on the condition, pain threshold as well as comfort level.

FREQUENCY AND DURATION

The frequency and duration of prostate milking can vary depending on health condition and the severity of symptoms.

Some of the methods and techniques commonly used include:

EXTERNAL MASSAGE

This is a non-invasive technique which involves massaging the perineum, the area between the scrotum and the anus, where the prostate can be indirectly stimulated. This method is less direct but can still help relieve symptoms and improve blood flow to the prostate gland.

INTERNAL MASSAGE

More direct than external massage, this method involves inserting a finger or a suitably sized dildo into the anus in order to apply gentle pressure to the prostate gland. This method allows for direct contact with the prostate and can be more effective in expelling stagnant secretions from the gland.

PROSTATE MASSAGERS

These are designed to match the anatomy of the prostate region and can be manually or battery-operated and are shaped to stimulate the prostate effectively and safely.

HYGIENE AND SAFETY

Keep in mind that maintaining high hygiene standards when performing internal prostate massages is important. Use gloves, adequate amounts of lubrication, and thoroughly clean tools to prevent infections.

HORMONAL CHANGES

In the prime of our youth, we experience the pinnacle of the hormone testosterone's influence, a period signified by a surge in sexual drive.

As we age, this hormonal high point gradually begins to wane, initiating a slow, inexorable decline where testosterone levels decrease by about 1% per year.

The decline in testosterone does not merely signify a reduction in sexual drive but also impacts muscle mass, bone density, and mood regulation. The body's lowered ability to produce testosterone can lead to a host of changes, including increased fatigue, a decrease in physical strength, and shifts in emotional well-being.

While challenging, this is a universal aspect of male aging. A holistic approach to health that encompasses diet, exercise, and possibly medical intervention can help you to manage and mitigate the multifaceted effects of reduced testosterone production.

For men with normal or lower than normal testosterone levels, the evidence of benefits from testosterone therapy to increase sexual desire and performance is less clear. Some studies have shown positive effects, while others have not found significant improvements.

Experiencing a decline in sex drive due to reduced hormonal production, especially testosterone, many can encounter a range of frustrations that affect both emotional and physical well-being.

LOSS OF IDENTITY

For many men, sexual prowess and the ability to maintain sexual activity are closely tied to their sense of masculinity and identity. A decrease in sex drive can lead some to feel like they are losing a part of what makes them "men," impacting their self-esteem and self-image.

RELATIONSHIP STRAIN

Some might feel frustrated or guilty if they believe they are no longer fulfilling their partner's sexual needs, possibly leading to tension and misunderstandings in relationships, especially if the situation is not openly discussed.

EMOTIONAL ISOLATION

The decline in sexual desire can lead to emotional withdrawal or feelings of isolation. Men might avoid discussing these changes due to embarrassment or fear of not being understood by their partners, friends, or family.

CONFUSION AND LACK OF INFORMATION

Many are not fully informed about the natural changes that come with aging. This lack of information can lead to confusion and misconceptions about what is normal, exacerbating feelings of anxiety and frustration. More on this topic in the chapter, **Creaky Cranky & Confused.**

DECREASED PHYSICAL SENSATION

Hormonal changes can affect not only the male sex drive, but also the physical pleasure derived from sexual activity. Some men may become frustrated by the decreased intensity of orgasms or the altered sensations during sexual encounters.

ERECTILE DYSFUNCTION

One of the more challenging aspects of decreased hormonal production can be erectile dysfunction (ED), which can impact a man's ability to engage in sexual activities. The frustration and embarrassment associated with ED can significantly affect a man's mental health and relationships.

FEAR OF AGING

A declining sex drive can serve as an unwelcome reminder of aging. Men might fear losing their youthfulness and vitality, leading to broader concerns about aging and mortality.

DEPRESSION AND ANXIETY

The cumulative impact of these aforementioned frustrations can lead to depression and anxiety. Some men might feel a persistent sadness or lose interest in activities they once enjoyed, increasing a sense of loss of life quality.

DECREASED SELF-CONFIDENCE

As sexual performance declines, so too can self-confidence. This can extend beyond intimate relationships into other areas of life that include social interactions and professional work.

RESISTANCE TO SEEK HELP

For some there is a reluctance to seek help because of associated stigma. This can delay addressing the issue, leading to prolonged frustration and a sense of helplessness.

Addressing the effects of reduced testosterone levels requires a multifaceted approach, including medical evaluation, counseling, open communication with partners, and sometimes lifestyle adjustments.

It's important to seek support and understand that these changes are a normal part of aging and how the natural diminution in testosterone production that comes with age can be further compounded by other factors including:

OBESITY

Excess body fat, especially around the waist, can disrupt hormone levels and lead to decreased testosterone production.

CHRONIC HEALTH CONDITIONS

Conditions like type 2 diabetes, kidney disease, and liver disease can affect hormone production.

MEDICATIONS

Certain medications, including opioids, steroids, and hormones used to treat prostate cancer as well as chemotherapy and radiation treatment can impact the body's natural testosterone production capabilities.

POOR DIET AND LACK OF EXERCISE

An unhealthy diet and lack of physical activity can negatively impact hormone levels, including testosterone.

CHRONIC STRESS

High levels of stress and the prolonged production of cortisol can lower testosterone levels.

SUBSTANCE ABUSE

Excessive alcohol consumption and the use of recreational drugs can negatively impact testosterone production.

SLEEP DISORDER

Poor sleep patterns and disorders like sleep apnea can reduce testosterone production

Though there are several reasons, physical and psychological, why our sex drive declines as we get older, many of which I have covered in this chapter, there are also plenty of reasons why keeping our libido active is beneficial to both our physiological health and our emotional well-being.

This chapter has hopefully reinforced the notion that aging and sexuality are not at odds with each other. They are instead intertwined in life's cycle of change. By embracing this, by staying healthy and communicative, I find myself not mourning youth as much as I celebrate it and welcome a mature perspective on getting older. Every phase of life offers its own unique pleasures and challenges, and that intimacy, in whatever form it takes, remains a vital part of the human experience regardless of age.

CHAPTER 9

The Aging Man's Survival Guide

DESIGNING RETIREMENT

Insights and inspiration to help you enjoy more of life after work.

The importance of having a well-rounded retirement plan in place post-60, focusing on financial considerations, lifestyle choices, climate, and relocation options, is the focus of this chapter. It also includes some of the benefits of moving abroad and a shortlist of countries that might provide a more comfortable and affordable retirement.

Whether or not you plan to work until your 70th birthday, once you have turned 60, the mental countdown to retirement will have likely already begun.

You can certainly walk past this milestone without much fanfare or even recognizing it as something to spend time dwelling on. Or, you can look at it soberly as a new and exciting chapter of your ongoing story. An era where living the best life you possibly can for the next 15 or so years should be in focus.

WHY JUST 15 YEARS?

Well, let's look at why. At 75 years of age, even if your mind is still young and agile, your body will more likely than not be perfectly happy to remind you regularly – and increasingly — that it's time to slow down. Not to mention that for every year we get older, the likelihood of past sins and/or genetic vulnerabilities catching up with us increases.

Once I turned 60, making plans to ensure that the next 15 or so years of my life were spent well made not only perfect sense healthwise, it became the only frame of mind I should reasonably have.

This is not to say that some will be perfectly happy with how things are and do not feel any need to change anything. That's fine, too. To each his/her own.

FUTURE PLANNING

For those of us who haven't had a retirement strategy in place before turning 60, it's not too late to start crafting one now. Not just a plan that considers our health and financial future. I'm talking about a thought-through, thorough strategy that ensures we get to enjoy as much of the rest of our active lives as possible.

First of all, I suggest thinking about and defining what's important and worth prioritizing. Is warm weather and an abundance of sunshine important and possibly a crucial component to your physical and mental health?

Do you have the financial means to maintain two homes and maybe even become a "Snowbird" during the year's chillier months?

Or, are you already living in a location where the weather is amazing regardless of season but you would like to travel a few times a year to either visit family and friends or discover new places and perhaps check off a few adventures from your bucket list?

Designing a solid retirement plan will not only give you peace of mind, the stability it can provide you with could be essential to maintaining independence as you age.

Here's a checklist to consider when designing your retirement:

FINANCIAL STABILITY

Assess your current financial situation, including savings, investments, and debts. Calculate how much you will need to cover your living expenses, factoring in inflation over the years.

Identify all potential sources of income during retirement, including Social Security benefits, pensions, retirement accounts (401(k), IRA), and any passive income sources like rental properties.

HEALTHCARE NEEDS

Plan for increasing healthcare costs, including Medicare, supplemental insurance, and potential long-term care. Consider investing in a health savings account (HSA) if eligible, to pay for medical expenses with pre-tax money.

LIFESTYLE GOALS

Define what you want your retirement to look like, including hobbies, travel, and time with family. Your goals will influence how much you need to save and how you allocate your resources.

HOUSING

Decide whether you'll downsize, relocate, or modify your current home to meet aging needs. Consider the costs of potential moves and home adaptations.

LONGEVITY RISK

Plan for a longer life expectancy to avoid outliving your savings. Consider annuities or other financial products that provide income for a longer than average life.

INFLATION

Accept that the cost of living will increase over time. Make sure your retirement income streams are structured to account for inflation, particularly in healthcare, food and housing.

TAX PLANNING

Understand how your investments, withdrawals, and Social Security benefits will be taxed. Structuring your withdrawals to minimize tax liabilities can extend the lifespan of your retirement funds.

ESTATE PLANNING

Arrange your estate affairs, including wills, trusts, and Power of Attorney. Ensure that your assets are protected and will be distributed according to your wishes. Read more on this topic in the epilogue, **Dealing with Denial & Mortality.**

EMERGENCY FUND

Maintain an emergency fund to cover unexpected expenses like major home repairs, healthcare needs, or family emergencies. This will help to protect your retirement savings from unforeseen expenses and withdrawals.

FOCUS ON LIVING COSTS

Budgeting for retirement can significantly enhance your financial security and, by extension, the quality of life you are focused on living. Prioritizing what's truly important to you and then gradually reducing indulgences, unnecessary purchases, and impulsive spending can make the shift to a lower income a whole lot smoother.

Decluttering your living space and selling items you no longer use can make downsizing or even relocating abroad much easier – as well as add money to your retirement fund.

When it comes to managing daily expenses during retirement, the approach can be pretty straightforward: after addressing fixed costs like housing, utilities, car payment and insurance, simply divide the remaining monthly funds you have by the number of days in the month.

This will be your daily budget. It's a simple strategy that not only discourages wasteful spending but also inspires savings for more meaningful, enriching experiences, like traveling.

MOVING & DOWNSIZING

Among the very first considerations during retirement planning is likely to be your disposable income in relation to your cost of living. Here you might want to think about downsizing your residential situation in order to achieve the lifestyle you yearn for as a retiree.

Relocating can provide both financial and practical upsides, as a new location might better align with your the life you want to lead.

Just by moving to a different part of town can offer lower living costs and other benefits. It's also important to consider factors like taxes, health care access and costs, as well as the overall economic climate of wherever you are thinking of moving to.

Most importantly, relocating to a new place that is more in line with your economic situation can add significant value to your retirement savings and by doing so, increase your financial stability. Exploring new environments, cultures, and communities, can be an enriching retirement experience in ways that wouldn't have been possible without relocating.

MOVING ABROAD

Exploring life in a new country can significantly broaden our horizons by offering exposure to different cultures, languages, and ways of life. On the practical side, many countries offer lower costs of living compared to Western Europe and the United States, allowing retirement savings to stretch further. Essentially, this can mean better access to healthcare, more comfortable housing, and being able to afford more leisure activities.

In addition to potential economic advantages, the adventure of adapting to a new environment and perhaps even learning a new language can also improve cognitive function, which is a significant benefit as we age.

Integrating into a new community can certainly be challenging, but it might also expand your social network, leading to meaningful relationships that might not have been possible if you had stayed in your home country.

Before making any definitive decisions, I recommend doing thorough research online and even making visits to considered places for relocation. Understanding the legal requirements for retiree residency and available visa options, healthcare alternatives, and the overall political and economical stability of the country are also important to think about.

It's also important to have an understanding of any tax implications moving abroad as a retiree might involve.

Contacting expatriates and online communities for those who have already made the move can provide you with valuable insights and help you avoid practical and financial pitfalls.

Embracing the challenge of moving abroad can lead to unexpected opportunities for personal growth. It encourages flexibility, resilience, and an open-minded approach to life's changes. Whether it's finding peace in a tranquil seaside village, immersing yourself in a bustling city's cultural scene, or simply enjoying a more relaxed pace of life, living abroad can dramatically enrich your retirement years.

Among countries generally considered both affordable and retirement-friendly are, in no particular order:

MEXICO

Mexico's reputation as a retirement haven is well-earned, with its inviting warm climate and rich tapestry of cultures drawing retirees from all corners of the globe. The country's affordability is particularly appealing, with lower living costs evident in its smaller towns and less touristy cities where one can enjoy a relaxed lifestyle without breaking the bank.

However, this cost-effectiveness can vary significantly; in Mexico's more sought-after locations, especially scenic coastal towns known for their expat communities, living expenses can climb, positioning these areas as less affordable options.

Despite this, even in these popular destinations, Mexico still offers a better cost of living compared to many parts of North America and Europe, blending cultural richness with economic practicality for retirees.

CAPITAL: Mexico City

FOUR MAJOR CITIES: Mexico City, Guadalajara, Monterrey, Puebla

PRIMARY LANGUAGE: Spanish

CURRENCY: Mexican Peso (MXN)

COUNTRY PHONE CODE: +52

MAJOR INDUSTRIES: Automotive, Electronics, Petroleum and Oil, Tourism, Agriculture

MAJOR EXPORTS: Vehicles, Electronic Equipment, Machinery, Oil and oil products, Silver, Fruits, Vegetables, Coffee, Cotton

TYPE OF GOVERNMENT: Federal Presidential Constitutional Republic

RETIREE VISA: Yes, Mexico offers a Temporary Resident Visa, suitable for retirees, which can be issued for up to 4 years, after which you may apply for permanent residency. Applicants must prove they have sufficient funds to sustain themselves or a steady income.

AVERAGE TEMPERATURE: Ranges significantly due to Mexico's varied topography. Coastal areas are typically warm with average temperatures ranging from 25°C to 28°C (77°F to 82°F), while higher elevations like Mexico City have cooler temperatures, averaging around 12°C to 16°C (53°F to 60°F).

POPULAR PLACES TO RELOCATE TO

PROS: Diverse choices including beach towns like Puerto Vallarta, cultural hubs like San Miguel de Allende, and temperate climates in cities like Guadalajara. Many areas have established expat communities offering a sense of belonging and resources for newcomers.

CONS: Popular areas may experience higher costs of living due to their desirability and influx of tourists.

COST OF LIVING

PROS: Generally lower than in many Western countries, enabling a comfortable lifestyle on a modest budget. Affordable real estate options, from renting to buying.

CONS: Tourist hotspots and expat-heavy regions might have inflated prices for housing and services.

INFRASTRUCTURE

PROS: Major cities and expat destinations offer modern amenities and infrastructure, including shopping centers, hospitals, and entertainment venues. Continuous improvements and investments in roads and public utilities.

CONS: Rural and less populated areas may lack reliable infrastructure and amenities.

UTILITIES

PROS: Utilities (electricity, water, internet) are generally cheaper compared to North American standards.

CONS: Service interruptions and reliability issues can occur, especially outside of major urban areas. Access to and Cost of Healthcare

PROS: High-quality healthcare available at significantly lower costs than in the U.S. Private healthcare is accessible and affordable. Many doctors and medical staff speak English, especially in cities and tourist areas.

CONS: Public healthcare facilities may be under-resourced and crowded. Remote areas might lack specialized medical services.

CLIMATE

PROS: Wide range of climates from tropical beaches to cooler highland areas, catering to all preferences. Mostly mild and pleasant weather in many parts of the country.

CONS: Some coastal areas can be extremely hot and humid, while highland regions may be cooler than preferred. Risk of hurricanes and earthquakes in certain regions.

FOOD

PROS: Fresh, flavorful, and diverse cuisine at low costs. Abundance of fresh produce year-round. Street food and local markets offer authentic and inexpensive eating options.

CONS: Adjusting to local food and water quality may take time for some expats. Risk of gastrointestinal issues initially.

ALCOHOL

PROS: Local beers, wines, and spirits like tequila and mezcal are of high quality and affordable. Lively bar and restaurant scene in urban and tourist areas.

CONS: Taxes on imported alcoholic beverages can make them more expensive.

SOCIAL LIFE

PROS: Friendly locals and a welcoming culture towards expats. Numerous social clubs, activities, and community groups geared towards retirees and expats.

CONS: Language barrier may limit initial social integration for those who do not speak Spanish.

CULTURE

PROS: Rich cultural heritage with numerous festivals, museums, and historical sites. Opportunity to learn Spanish and immerse in a vibrant cultural setting.

CONS: Cultural and bureaucratic differences can be challenging to navigate without local knowledge or language skills.

TRANSPORTATION

PROS: Affordable public transportation options in cities. Taxis and ride-sharing services are widely available. Growing network of high-quality roads and highways.

CONS: Traffic congestion in major cities. Rural areas may have limited transportation options.

CAR HIRE AND FUEL

PROS: Car rental and fuel costs are reasonable, facilitating travel and exploration.

CONS: Traffic laws and driving habits may differ from what expats are accustomed to, posing challenges.

INTERNET ACCESS

PROS: Good internet connectivity in urban and popular expat areas, with competitive pricing for services.

CONS: Internet speed and reliability may be inconsistent in rural or remote locations.

SAFETY

PROS: Many expat communities and tourist areas are safe and have low crime rates.

CONS: Concerns about crime and safety persist in certain areas, especially related to drug cartel activity.

JUDICIAL

PROS: Access to legal resources and services for expats.

CONS: Legal processes can be slow and complicated by bureaucracy.

POLITICAL STABILITY

PROS: Mexico has a stable political system with regular, democratic elections.

CONS: Political and economic reforms can lead to uncertainty and protests, potentially affecting expats.

PANAMA

Panama's allure for retirees extends beyond its tropical climate to encompass a range of financial and lifestyle benefits, particularly through its Pensionado Visa program. This program is specifically designed to attract retirees from around the world, offering them substantial discounts on essential and leisure services.

These incentives include significant savings on healthcare services, which is a major consideration for many retirees, as well as on entertainment options and transportation, making daily living and enjoyment of the country's vast cultural and natural offerings more affordable.

The discounts provided under the Pensionado Visa make Panama an even more attractive destination for retirees seeking a comfortable and economically viable lifestyle in their later years, allowing them to stretch their retirement savings further while enjoying the lifestyle Panama offers.

CAPITAL: Panama City

FOUR MAJOR CITIES: Panama City, San Miguelito, David, La Chorrera

PRIMARY LANGUAGE: Spanish

CURRENCY: Balboa (PAB) and U.S. Dollar (USD) are both officially used.

COUNTRY PHONE CODE: +507

MAJOR INDUSTRIES: Banking, Commerce, Tourism, Trading, Shipping (due to the Panama Canal)

MAJOR EXPORTS: Fruits (mainly bananas), seafood, iron and steel waste, gold, and coffee

TYPE OF GOVERNMENT: Unitary presidential constitutional republic

RETIREE VISA: Yes, Panama offers the Pensionado Visa, available to anyone with a lifetime pension of at least $1,000 per month. It provides discounts on services and goods, including medical services, entertainment, flights, and utility bills.

AVERAGE TEMPERATURE: The temperature in Panama is fairly consistent year-round, with averages ranging from 24°C to 29°C (75°F to 84°F) due to its tropical climate.

POPULAR PLACES TO RELOCATE TO

PROS: Boquete, Coronado, and Panama City offer vibrant expat communities, beautiful landscapes, and ample amenities. Diverse options ranging from beachfront communities to mountainous retreats cater to varied preferences.

CONS: Some popular areas may become overcrowded or lose their charm due to rapid development and increased living costs.

COST OF LIVING

PROS: Generally lower than in the US and Canada, especially outside of Panama City. Pensionado program offers significant discounts to retirees on a range of services and utilities.

CONS: Cost of living in Panama City and other expat hotspots can be high, comparable to or even exceeding prices in North America.

INFRASTRUCTURE

PROS: Modern infrastructure in urban areas, including shopping centers, hospitals, and roads. Significant investments in public transportation, including the Panama Metro in Panama City.

CONS: Infrastructure quality and reliability can drop significantly in rural or less developed areas.

UTILITIES

PROS: Utilities are generally reliable and affordable in urban and popular expat areas.

CONS: In remote areas, utilities like electricity and water can be less reliable, with occasional outages.

ACCESS TO AND COST OF HEALTHCARE

PROS: High-quality healthcare available at a fraction of US costs in major cities. Many doctors are US-trained, and private hospitals offer excellent care.

CONS: Public healthcare facilities may be overcrowded and under-resourced.

Health insurance and private healthcare can be expensive for those with pre-existing conditions.

CLIMATE

PROS: Tropical climate with warm weather year-round in most of the country.

Cooler temperatures in the highlands, offering a comfortable climate for those who prefer milder weather.

CONS: High humidity and heat in coastal areas can be uncomfortable for some. Rainy season can bring heavy rainfall and flooding in certain areas.

FOOD

PROS: Fresh tropical fruits, vegetables, and seafood are widely available and affordable. Panamanian cuisine is diverse and flavorful, influenced by a mix of cultures.

CONS: Imported food products and international cuisine can be pricey.

ALCOHOL

PROS: Local beers, rum, and other spirits are affordable. Wine and imported spirits are available but may be more expensive.

CONS: Taxes on alcohol can make imported drinks costly.

SOCIAL LIFE

PROS: Welcoming expat communities and friendly locals make it easy to build a social network.

Wide variety of social activities, clubs, and groups catering to diverse interests.

CONS: Language barrier may limit social interactions with locals for non-Spanish speakers.

CULTURE

PROS: Rich cultural heritage with influences from Indigenous, Latin American, Caribbean, and European traditions. Vibrant music, dance, and festival scene.

CONS: Cultural differences and language barrier may pose challenges for deeper integration.

TRANSPORTATION

PROS: Affordable public transportation options in urban areas, including buses and metro. Panama City's Tocumen International Airport offers good international connectivity.

CONS: Traffic congestion in Panama City can be severe. In rural areas, public transportation options are limited and less reliable.

CAR HIRE AND FUEL

PROS: Car rental services are widely available and reasonably priced. Fuel prices are generally lower than in North America and Europe.

CONS: Traffic and driving practices may be challenging for newcomers.

INTERNET ACCESS

PROS: Good internet coverage and high-speed options available in urban and popular expat areas.

CONS: Internet service can be unreliable and slower in rural or remote locations.

SAFETY

PROS: Many parts of Panama are safe and have low crime rates, especially in expat communities and rural areas.

CONS: Certain areas, particularly in and around some parts of Panama City, have higher crime rates, including petty theft and violent crime.

JUDICIAL

PROS: Legal assistance and services are accessible for expats.

CONS: The judicial system can be slow, and legal proceedings can be prolonged and complicated.

POLITICAL STABILITY

PROS: Panama has a stable political environment with a democratic government structure.

CONS: Political demonstrations and protests, while generally peaceful, can occasionally disrupt daily activities and services.

PORTUGAL

Portugal offers an idyllic setting for retirees seeking a blend of European charm and affordable living. Its mild climate ensures comfortable temperatures year-round, perfect for enjoying the country's extensive coastline and lush interiors.

With its rich cultural heritage, evident in its historic cities, traditional villages, and numerous festivals, Portugal provides a deep sense of connection to the past while embracing modern comforts and conveniences. Particularly in smaller towns, the cost of living allows retirees to enjoy a comfortable life without the financial strain found in many other Western European countries.

This combination of climate, culture, and affordability makes Portugal an appealing option for those looking to enrich their retirement years with new experiences and a relaxed lifestyle.

CAPITAL: Lisbon

FOUR MAJOR CITIES: Lisbon, Porto, Braga, Faro

PRIMARY LANGUAGE: Portuguese

CURRENCY: Euro (EUR)

COUNTRY PHONE CODE: +351

MAJOR INDUSTRIES: Tourism, Textiles, Clothing, Footwear, Cork and Cork products, Wine, Technology, and Automobiles.

MAJOR EXPORTS: Vehicles, electrical machinery, mineral fuels, pharmaceuticals, and footwear.

TYPE OF GOVERNMENT: Semi-presidential representative democratic republic

RETIREE VISA: Yes, Portugal offers a D7 Visa, often referred to as the Retirement or Passive Income Visa, designed for retirees or people with a stable passive income.

AVERAGE TEMPERATURE: Varies from 12°C in the north to 18°C in the south. The Algarve region enjoys mild winters and warm summers.

SPECIFIC AND POPULAR PLACES TO RELOCATE TO

PROS: Lisbon, Porto, the Algarve, and Madeira are popular, offering vibrant cultural scenes and beautiful landscapes.

CONS: These areas can be more expensive due to their popularity and might not provide an authentic Portuguese living experience due to the high number of expats and tourists.

COST OF LIVING

PROS: Generally lower than in many Western European countries, especially in rural areas.

CONS: Popular expat destinations like Lisbon and the Algarve have seen a significant increase in living costs.

INFRASTRUCTURE

PROS: Good public transport in cities, well-maintained roads, and high-speed internet widely available.

CONS: Rural areas may lack some modern infrastructures, like reliable internet and public transportation.

UTILITIES

PROS: Utilities are generally affordable.

CONS: Electricity prices are high compared to the EU average.

ACCESS TO AND COST OF HEALTHCARE

PROS: High-quality healthcare services; lower healthcare costs than in many other Western countries.

CONS: Public healthcare system can experience long wait times for certain procedures and services.

CLIMATE

PROS: Mild, Mediterranean climate with hot summers and wet, mild winters in most regions.

CONS: Northern regions experience more rainfall and colder temperatures, which may not appeal to everyone.

FOOD

PROS: Fresh, high-quality, and diverse cuisine at reasonable prices.

CONS: Smaller towns and rural areas may lack international cuisine options.

ALCOHOL

PROS: Excellent quality wine and spirits at very affordable prices.

CONS: Heavy drinking culture might not suit everyone.

SOCIAL LIFE

PROS: Warm and welcoming locals, easy to make friends, and a strong sense of community.

CONS: Language barrier might limit social interactions initially.

CULTURE

PROS: Rich historical and cultural heritage with numerous festivals, museums, and events.

CONS: Adjustment to local customs and slower pace of life may take time for some.

TRANSPORTATION

PROS: Extensive and affordable public transport network in urban areas.

CONS: Rural areas often require a car due to less frequent public transport services.

CAR HIRE AND FUEL

PROS: Car rental services are widely available and reasonably priced.

CONS: High fuel costs compared to some other countries.

INTERNET ACCESS

PROS: High-speed internet is widely available at competitive prices.

CONS: Rural areas might have limited options and slower speeds.

SAFETY

PROS: Portugal is one of the safest countries in the world with low crime rates.

CONS: Petty crime like pickpocketing can be an issue in tourist areas.

JUDICIAL

PROS: EU member state with a well-established legal framework.

CONS: Judicial processes can be slow, and navigating the legal system can be challenging for expats.

POLITICAL STABILITY

PROS: Portugal enjoys a stable political environment with a low risk of political violence.

CONS: Bureaucracy and economic challenges can lead to public dissatisfaction and protests.

MALAYSIA

This Southeast Asian nation is known for its affordable healthcare, diverse culture, and beautiful landscapes.

CAPITAL: Kuala Lumpur

FOUR MAJOR CITIES: Kuala Lumpur, George Town (Penang), Johor Bahru, Ipoh

PRIMARY LANGUAGE: Malay (Bahasa Melayu)

CURRENCY: Malaysian Ringgit (MYR)

COUNTRY PHONE CODE: +60

MAJOR INDUSTRIES: Electronics, petroleum and liquefied natural gas production, palm oil, and rubber production.

MAJOR EXPORTS: Electrical and electronic products, petroleum and liquefied natural gas, palm oil, and rubber.

TYPE OF GOVERNMENT: Federal constitutional monarchy with a parliamentary democracy

RETIREE VISA: Yes, Malaysia offers the Malaysia My Second Home (MM2H) programme, which allows foreigners to live in Malaysia on a long-term basis.

AVERAGE TEMPERATURE: Ranges between 23°C to 32°C throughout the year.

SPECIFIC AND POPULAR PLACES TO RELOCATE TO

PROS: Kuala Lumpur for city life, Penang for cultural heritage and cuisine, Langkawi for beaches and natural beauty, and the Cameron Highlands for cooler climates and tea plantations.

CONS: Popular areas can be more expensive and crowded, particularly Kuala Lumpur and Penang.

COST OF LIVING

PROS: Generally lower than in Western countries, with affordable housing, food, and services.

CONS: Expatriate areas and popular tourist destinations have higher living costs.

INFRASTRUCTURES

PROS: Well-developed in major cities with good healthcare, transportation, and telecommunications.

CONS: Rural areas may lack the same level of infrastructure quality and reliability.

UTILITIES

PROS: Utilities (electricity, water, internet) are generally affordable.

CONS: Occasional disruptions in utilities services can occur, especially in less urbanized areas.

ACCESS TO AND COST OF HEALTHCARE

PROS: High-quality healthcare facilities in major cities; healthcare costs are reasonable.

CONS: Rural areas may have limited access to advanced medical care.

CLIMATE

PROS: Warm, tropical climate year-round.

CONS: High humidity and frequent rainfall; air quality can be poor during haze episodes.

FOOD

PROS: Diverse and flavorful cuisine with a mix of Malay, Chinese, Indian, and international dishes.

CONS: Dietary restrictions (e.g., gluten-free, vegan) may be harder to accommodate in traditional eateries.

ALCOHOL

PROS: Available in urban areas and tourist spots.

CONS: Relatively expensive due to high taxes; less accessible in predominantly Muslim areas due to religious reasons.

SOCIAL LIFE

PROS: Malaysians are generally warm and welcoming; expatriate communities are active.

CONS: Language and cultural differences can pose initial barriers to social integration.

CULTURE

PROS: Rich cultural diversity offering a mix of Malay, Chinese, Indian, and indigenous cultures.

CONS: Conservative social norms may require adjustment for those from more liberal countries.

TRANSPORTATION

PROS: Comprehensive public transportation in major cities; affordable taxis and ride-hailing services.

CONS: Traffic congestion in urban areas; public transport options may be limited in rural regions.

CAR HIRE AND FUEL

PROS: Fuel prices are relatively low; car rental options are widely available.

CONS: Traffic congestion in cities; some rural areas have challenging road conditions.

INTERNET ACCESS

PROS: High-speed internet is widely available in urban and suburban areas at competitive prices.

CONS: Internet service can be less reliable and slower in rural or remote areas.

SAFETY

PROS: Generally safe for expatriates; low rates of violent crime.

CONS: Petty crime (e.g., theft, scams) can be a concern in tourist-heavy areas.

JUDICIAL

PROS: Legal system based on British common law; specialized courts for commercial, family, and administrative matters.

CONS: Legal processes can be slow, and there have been concerns about judicial independence.

POLITICAL STABILITY

PROS: Malaysia has a history of political stability with peaceful transitions of power.

CONS: Political landscape can be complex with occasional tensions and shifts in alliances.

COLOMBIA

Colombia offers a mix of vibrant cities and picturesque countryside, with a low cost of living that makes the country particularly appealing.

CAPITAL: Bogotá

FOUR MAJOR CITIES: Medellín, Cali, Barranquilla, Cartagena

PRIMARY LANGUAGE: Spanish

CURRENCY: Colombian Peso (COP)

COUNTRY PHONE CODE: +57

MAJOR INDUSTRIES: Oil, mining (coal, gold, and emeralds), textiles, clothing, and footwear, beverages, agriculture (coffee, flowers, bananas, and cut flowers).

MAJOR EXPORTS: Petroleum, coffee, coal, nickel, emeralds, apparel, bananas, cut flowers.

TYPE OF GOVERNMENT: Unitary presidential constitutional republic

RETIREE VISA: Yes, Colombia offers a retirement visa, known as a "Pensionado Visa," which requires proof of a minimum monthly income from a pension or retirement fund.

AVERAGE TEMPERATURE: Varies widely due to altitude and geography but generally ranges from 14°C in Bogotá to 28°C in Cartagena.

RELOCATION CONSIDERATIONS

SPECIFIC AND POPULAR PLACES TO RELOCATE TO

PROS: Medellín (eternal spring climate, innovative city), Cartagena (historic, Caribbean coast), Cali (salsa capital, warm), Santa Marta (beaches, nature).

CONS: Larger cities can be congested; some coastal areas are prone to humidity and heat.

COST OF LIVING

PROS: Generally lower than in the US and Europe, affordable housing, food, and services.

CONS: Popular expat areas might have inflated prices.

INFRASTRUCTURE

PROS: Major cities have good healthcare, public transportation, and modern amenities.

CONS: Rural and remote areas may lack reliable infrastructure and services.

UTILITIES

PROS: Utilities are reasonably priced in most areas.

CONS: Occasional service interruptions; rural areas might have less reliable access.

ACCESS TO AND COST OF HEALTHCARE

PROS: High-quality healthcare available in major cities; lower costs compared to North America and Europe.

CONS: Access can be limited in more remote areas; public hospitals might have longer waiting times.

CLIMATE

PROS: Diverse climates, from warm coastal regions to cooler Andean highlands.

CONS: Certain areas are prone to heavy rainfall or high humidity.

FOOD

PROS: Rich culinary traditions, fresh tropical fruits, and affordable dining options.

CONS: Some international cuisine options might be limited outside major cities.

ALCOHOL

PROS: Locally produced beers and spirits are affordable.

CONS: Imported alcohol can be costly.

SOCIAL LIFE

PROS: Colombians are known for their warmth and hospitality; vibrant music and dance scene.

CONS: Language barrier might limit social interactions initially.

CULTURE

PROS: Rich cultural heritage, festivals, and traditions; significant historical sites.

CONS: Adjusting to local customs and schedules may take time for some.

TRANSPORTATION

PROS: Affordable public transportation options in cities; diverse terrain accessible by road.

CONS: Traffic congestion in cities; rural areas might have less frequent services.

CAR HIRE AND FUEL

PROS: Car rentals are available; fuel prices are reasonable.

CONS: Traffic in urban areas; challenging driving conditions in rural regions.

INTERNET ACCESS

PROS: Good internet access in urban areas at reasonable prices.

CONS: Internet reliability decreases in rural and remote locations.

SAFETY

PROS: Significant improvements in safety and security in recent years.

CONS: Some areas still have high crime rates; caution advised in certain regions.

JUDICIAL

PROS: Legal reforms and efforts to improve the judicial system.

CONS: Slow legal processes and concerns over impartiality.

POLITICAL STABILITY

PROS: Recent years have seen a move towards greater stability and peace.

CONS: Historical political tensions and ongoing negotiations with rebel groups.

THAILAND

Thailand offers a compelling blend of breathtaking natural beauty, from its pristine beaches and lush jungles to its vibrant cities and historical temples, making it a sought-after destination not only for tourists but also for expatriates and retirees.

Beyond its scenic allure and deep cultural heritage, the country is attractive for its affordability. The cost of living in Thailand is relatively low, allowing for a comfortable lifestyle that includes dining out, entertainment, and travel within a modest budget.

Additionally, Thailand boasts an excellent healthcare system, recognized for its high-quality medical services, modern facilities, and well-trained healthcare professionals, all at a fraction of the cost compared to Western countries. This combination of factors makes Thailand an ideal place for those seeking a blend of comfort, and wellness.

CAPITAL: Bangkok

FOUR MAJOR CITIES: Bangkok, Chiang Mai, Phuket Town, and Pattaya

PRIMARY LANGUAGE: Thai

CURRENCY: Thai Baht (THB)

COUNTRY PHONE CODE: +66

MAJOR INDUSTRIES: Tourism, textiles and garments, agricultural processing, beverages, tobacco, cement, light manufacturing including jewelry and electric appliances, computers and parts, integrated circuits, furniture, automobiles and automotive parts.

MAJOR EXPORTS: Computers and parts, cars and automotive parts, electrical appliances, machinery and equipment, textiles and footwear, fishery products, rice, rubber.

TYPE OF GOVERNMENT: Constitutional monarchy with a parliamentary system.

RETIREE VISA: Thailand offers a retirement visa for foreigners over the age of 50, known as the "Non-Immigrant O-A Long Stay Visa," which is valid for one year and renewable.

AVERAGE TEMPERATURE: Ranges from 18°C to 38°C (64°F to 100°F), depending on the season and region.

PROS AND CONS OF RELOCATING TO THAILAND

SPECIFIC AND POPULAR PLACES TO RELOCATE TO

PROS: Thailand offers a variety of attractive locations for expatriates, including bustling Bangkok for urban life, Chiang Mai for culture and cooler climate, Phuket and Pattaya for beach life, and Hua Hin for a quiet seaside town.

CONS: Some areas, especially in popular tourist destinations, can be overcrowded and more expensive due to their popularity.

COST OF LIVING

PROS: Generally lower than in many Western countries, especially in terms of food, local transportation, and services.

CONS: Costs in touristy areas and for imported goods can be high; the cost of living in Bangkok is significantly higher than in other parts of the country.

INFRASTRUCTURE

PROS: Good infrastructure in major cities, including modern airports, public transportation systems, and healthcare facilities.

CONS: Rural areas may lack the same level of infrastructure, with less reliable roads and public services.

UTILITIES

PROS: Generally affordable, especially water and electricity.

CONS: Occasional issues with reliability in certain areas, and air conditioning can significantly increase electricity bills due to the hot climate.

ACCESS TO AND COST OF HEALTHCARE

PROS: High-quality healthcare available in major cities, with English-speaking staff in many private hospitals.

CONS: Healthcare in rural areas may not meet the standards of major cities; private healthcare can be expensive without insurance.

CLIMATE

PROS: Warm, tropical climate year-round.

CONS: High humidity and heat can be uncomfortable; monsoon season brings heavy rains.

FOOD

PROS: Delicious, diverse cuisine at affordable prices. Availability of international foods in cities is outstanding.

CONS: Those unaccustomed to spicy food may need time to adjust.

ALCOHOL

PROS: Widely available, with a good selection of local and international brands.

CONS: Alcohol taxes can make some imported drinks expensive

SOCIAL LIFE

PROS: Vibrant expat communities and friendly locals make it easy to meet people; numerous social, cultural, and outdoor activities.

CONS: Language barrier can limit deeper integration into Thai society for those not fluent in Thai.

CULTURE

PROS: Rich and accessible Thai culture, with countless temples, festivals, and traditions to explore.

CONS: Cultural differences and language barriers may lead to misunderstandings.

TRANSPORTATION

PROS: Extensive and affordable public transportation options in cities; easy to find taxis and ride-sharing services.

CONS: Periodic traffic congestion in cities like Bangkok and Chiang Mai.

CAR HIRE AND FUEL

PROS: Car rental and fuel are reasonably priced by international standards.

CONS: Driving in urban Thai cities can be challenging due to traffic conditions and different driving habits and the fact that they drive on the left side of the road.

INTERNET ACCESS

PROS: Good internet access in urban areas, with competitive pricing for high-speed connections.

CONS: Internet reliability can be an issue in more remote areas.

POLITICAL STABILITY:

Thailand has a strong sense of national identity and a long history of political stability.

SAFETY:

Safe for expatriates and tourists with low crime rates.

COSTA RICA

Costa Rica stands out as a gem in Central America, admired not only for its lush rainforests, stunning coastlines, and diverse wildlife but also for its appealing cost of living.

Particularly away from the more tourist-centric locales, expats find that their dollars stretch further, affording a comfortable and enjoyable lifestyle amidst the country's natural splendor.

Markets brimming with fresh, local produce, affordable healthcare, and modest housing costs contribute to the appeal, making Costa Rica an attractive destination for expatriates and retirees seeking a tranquil, eco-friendly lifestyle without the hefty price tag often associated with such pristine environments.

This balance of natural beauty and affordability makes Costa Rica an ideal choice for those wishing to live in harmony with nature while maintaining a cost-effective lifestyle.

CAPITAL: San José

FOUR MAJOR CITIES: Alajuela, Cartago, Heredia, Limón

PRIMARY LANGUAGE: Spanish

CURRENCY: Costa Rican Colón (CRC)

COUNTRY PHONE CODE: +506

MAJOR INDUSTRIES: Tourism, agriculture, microprocessors, medical equipment, electronic components.

MAJOR EXPORTS: Medical instruments, bananas, pineapples, coffee, and ornamental plants.

TYPE OF GOVERNMENT: Democratic Republic

RETIREE VISA: Costa Rica offers a "Pensionado" visa for retirees who can prove a minimum monthly income of $1,000 from a pension or retirement fund.

AVERAGE TEMPERATURE: Varies widely depending on altitude and area, but generally ranges between 18°C (64°F) in the highlands to 27°C (81°F) in the lowlands.

SPECIFIC AND POPULAR PLACES TO RELOCATE TO

PROS: Expat favorites include the Central Valley for its mild climate, the Pacific Coast for its beaches and expat communities, and the Northern Plains for its natural beauty.

CONS: Some popular areas can be more expensive due to demand from foreigners and tourists.

COST OF LIVING

PROS: Generally lower than in the US and Canada, especially for local products and services.

CONS: Imported goods, luxury items, and certain services can be expensive.

INFRASTRUCTURE

PROS: Good in major cities and popular expat areas, with reliable services and amenities.

CONS: Rural areas may lack quality infrastructure, including roads, which can be challenging, especially in the rainy season.

UTILITIES

PROS: Basic utilities (water, electricity) are generally reliable and affordable in urban areas.

CONS: Electricity can be costly, particularly for those using air conditioning or heating due to the varied climate.

ACCESS TO AND COST OF HEALTHCARE

PROS: High-quality healthcare available at both public and private facilities; costs are lower than in the US.

CONS: Public healthcare may involve long waits; private healthcare, while faster, is more expensive.

CLIMATE

PROS: Diverse climate zones offer options for everyone; from tropical beaches to temperate mountains.

CONS: The rainy season can be intense, affecting mobility and outdoor activities.

FOOD

PROS: Fresh, local produce is widely available and inexpensive; diverse international cuisine in urban areas.

CONS: Imported food items can be costly.

ALCOHOL

PROS: Local beers, spirits, and wines are readily available at reasonable prices.

CONS: Imported alcoholic beverages are subject to high taxes, making them expensive.

SOCIAL LIFE

PROS: Friendly locals and a significant expat community make it easy to build an engaging social life.

CONS: Language barrier can be an issue for non-Spanish speakers, potentially limiting deeper interactions with locals.

CULTURE

PROS: Rich in biodiversity and culture, offering numerous festivals, museums, and historical sites.

CONS: Cultural adjustment can take time for expats, including adapting to the laid-back approach to time and schedules.

TRANSPORTATION

PROS: Comprehensive public transportation network in urban areas; affordable domestic flights.

CONS: Traffic congestion in cities; road conditions in rural areas can be poor.

CAR HIRE AND FUEL

PROS: Car rental options are plentiful, with competitive pricing.

CONS: High fuel costs; driving can be challenging due to aggressive local driving styles and road conditions.

INTERNET ACCESS

PROS: Good internet coverage and speed in urban and popular expat areas; competitive pricing.

CONS: Internet service can be unreliable and slower in remote or rural areas.

SAFETY

PROS: Generally considered safe for tourists and expats, with a lower crime rate than other Latin American countries.

CONS: Petty crimes, mostly theft and burglary, do occur, especially in tourist areas.

JUDICIAL

PROS: Legal system is accessible; property rights are well respected.

CONS: Bureaucracy can be slow; legal processes may be lengthy and complex for foreigners.

POLITICAL STABILITY

PROS: Costa Rica is known for its political stability, absence of a standing army, and peaceful democratic governance.

CONS: Like any country, political changes and debates, especially regarding fiscal policy and social issues, can create uncertainty.

VIETNAM

Vietnam stands out as a prime retirement destination, offering an enticing combination of affordability, rich cultural history, and stunningly diverse landscapes. From the bustling streets of Hanoi and Ho Chi Minh City to the serene beauty of Ha Long Bay and the rolling hills of Sapa, Vietnam provides a backdrop that caters to a wide range of interests and lifestyles.

The cost of living is remarkably low, allowing retirees to enjoy a comfortable lifestyle with access to high-quality healthcare, housing, and fresh, flavorful cuisine at a fraction of the cost compared to many Western countries.

Vietnam's deep historical roots, visible in its ancient temples, colonial architecture, and vibrant cultural festivals, offer great opportunities for exploration and discovery, making it not just a place to live but a place to experience with all senses.

CAPITAL: Hanoi

FOUR MAJOR CITIES: Ho Chi Minh City, Da Nang, Hai Phong, Can Tho

PRIMARY LANGUAGE: Vietnamese

CURRENCY: Vietnamese Dong (VND)

COUNTRY PHONE CODE: +84

MAJOR INDUSTRIES: Electronics, textiles and garments, footwear, agriculture, fishery, and tourism.

MAJOR EXPORTS: Electronics, textiles, clothing, footwear, coffee, rice, seafood, and wooden products.

TYPE OF GOVERNMENT: Socialist Republic

RETIREE VISA: Vietnam offers a visa exemption for certain nationalities and visa-on-arrival or e-visa for others, but there is no specific retirement visa. Long-term stay requires periodic renewal of visas.

AVERAGE TEMPERATURE: Ranges from 22°C in the north to up to 27°C in the south, with variations in climate zones.

Specific and Popular Places to Relocate to

PROS: Expats often choose vibrant Ho Chi Minh City for its dynamic lifestyle, Hanoi for its blend of traditional and modern cultures, Da Nang for its coastal living, and Hoi An for its historic charm and slower pace of life.

CONS: Urban centers can be crowded and noisy, while more scenic locations might lack some modern amenities.

COST OF LIVING

PROS: Generally low, especially for local goods and services, allowing for a comfortable lifestyle on a modest budget.

CONS: Costs in expat-popular areas and for imported goods can be higher than the local average.

INFRASTRUCTURE

PROS: Rapid improvements in urban areas with modern facilities and services.

CONS: Some rural and remote areas still have underdeveloped infrastructure.

UTILITIES

PROS: Utilities like electricity, water, and gas are relatively inexpensive.

CONS: Occasional power outages and water shortages can occur, especially in less developed areas.

ACCESS TO AND COST OF HEALTHCARE

PROS: Affordable healthcare services with several international hospitals in major cities.

CONS: Healthcare quality can be inconsistent outside of major urban centers; language barriers may exist.

CLIMATE

PROS: Varied climate zones offer a choice between tropical and temperate weather conditions.

CONS: The country experiences a monsoon season, which can lead to heavy rainfall and flooding in certain areas.

FOOD

PROS: Diverse, flavorful, and affordable cuisine with a wide variety of local and international options.

CONS: Dietary restrictions or preferences (e.g., gluten-free, vegan) might be harder to accommodate outside major cities.

ALCOHOL

PROS: Local beers and spirits are widely available and inexpensive.

CONS: Imported alcoholic beverages can be costly due to taxes.

SOCIAL LIFE

PROS: Vibrant expat communities and friendly locals facilitate an active social life.

CONS: Cultural and language barriers can pose challenges to deeper integration with local communities.

CULTURE

PROS: Rich cultural heritage with numerous festivals, traditions, and historical sites to explore.

CONS: Adjusting to local customs and etiquette may require time and effort for newcomers.

TRANSPORTATION

PROS: Affordable public transport options in cities, along with cheap taxi and motorbike services.

CONS: Traffic congestion is a significant issue in major cities, and road safety standards can be a concern.

CAR HIRE AND FUEL

PROS: Car and motorbike rentals are readily available for exploring.

CONS: High costs of car ownership and fuel, along with challenging driving conditions.

INTERNET ACCESS

PROS: Good internet connectivity in urban areas with competitive pricing.

CONS: Internet service can be less reliable and slower in rural or remote locations.

SAFETY

PROS: Vietnam is generally safe for expats and tourists, with low violent crime rates.

CONS: Petty crimes like theft and scams targeting foreigners can occur, especially in tourist areas.

JUDICIAL

PROS: Legal processes and systems are in place for dispute resolution.

CONS: The judicial system can be slow and difficult to navigate for foreigners, with concerns about transparency.

POLITICAL STABILITY

PROS: Vietnam has enjoyed a period of political stability, contributing to economic growth.

CONS: The country's one-party political system has some restrictions.

GREECE

Greece, with its idyllic warm Mediterranean climate, beckons those seeking a life full of sunshine and characterized by mild winters and hot, dry summers. Beyond its weather, Greece is particularly appealing for its affordable cost of living, especially noticeable in smaller towns and islands away from the bustling cities like Athens and Thessaloniki.

These less populous locales offer a serene lifestyle amidst ancient ruins, stunning landscapes, and crystal-clear waters, all while maintaining a lower cost of living.

This affordability extends to daily expenses, from fresh, locally-sourced food to property costs, making Greece an attractive destination for retirees, expats, and anyone dreaming of a life in a picturesque setting that combines history, culture, and natural beauty with economic practicality.

CAPITAL: Athens

FOUR MAJOR CITIES: Thessaloniki, Patras, Heraklion, Larissa

PRIMARY LANGUAGE: Greek

CURRENCY: Euro (EUR)

COUNTRY PHONE CODE: +30

MAJOR INDUSTRIES: Tourism, shipping, agriculture, and manufacturing.

MAJOR EXPORTS: Olive oil, fruits and vegetables, yogurt, cheese, pharmaceuticals, and textiles.

TYPE OF GOVERNMENT: Parliamentary Republic

RETIREE VISA: Greece offers a residence permit for financially independent persons, allowing non-EU retirees to live in Greece if they meet certain income requirements.

AVERAGE TEMPERATURE: Varies from Mediterranean to continental climates; coastal areas enjoy mild winters and hot, dry summers, while inland areas have colder winters.

SPECIFIC AND POPULAR PLACES TO RELOCATE TO

PROS: Popular relocation destinations include the idyllic islands of Crete, Rhodes, and Corfu, offering beautiful landscapes and a slower pace of life, as well as Athens for those seeking a vibrant urban environment.

CONS: Tourist hotspots can be crowded and more expensive, especially in summer.

COST OF LIVING

PROS: Generally lower than many Western European countries, especially in smaller towns and rural areas.

CONS: Living costs in popular islands and cities like Athens can be higher due to tourism and demand.

INFRASTRUCTURE

PROS: Good infrastructure in major cities and tourist areas, including healthcare, transportation, and services.

CONS: Some remote areas and smaller islands may have less developed infrastructure.

UTILITIES

PROS: Utility costs (water, electricity, gas) are generally reasonable.

CONS: Electricity can be expensive, especially in peak summer months due to air conditioning use.

ACCESS TO AND COST OF HEALTHCARE

PROS: High standard of public healthcare available at low cost; private healthcare is also affordable and offers shorter waiting times.

CONS: Rural areas might lack immediate access to advanced healthcare facilities.

CLIMATE

PROS: Warm Mediterranean climate with abundant sunshine, mild winters, and hot summers.

CONS: Summers can be excessively hot, especially in cities and on some islands.

FOOD

PROS: Fresh, locally-produced food is widely available and affordable; Greek cuisine is diverse and flavorful.

CONS: International cuisine options may be limited in smaller towns and rural areas.

ALCOHOL

PROS: Local wines and spirits are of high quality and reasonably priced.

CONS: Imported alcoholic beverages can be expensive.

SOCIAL LIFE

PROS: Greeks are known for their hospitality; expats can enjoy a rich social life and community.

CONS: Language barriers may exist, although many Greeks speak English, especially in urban and tourist areas.

CULTURE

PROS: Rich historical and cultural heritage, with numerous sites, traditions, and festivals.

CONS: Adjusting to the relaxed pace of life can at times be challenging.

TRANSPORTATION

PROS: Comprehensive public transportation network in cities; numerous options for domestic travel.

CONS: Rural areas may have limited public transport options; islands may require travel by boat.

CAR HIRE AND FUEL

PROS: Car hire is widely available and provides flexibility for exploration.

CONS: Fuel prices are high; driving in cities can be challenging due to traffic and parking.

INTERNET ACCESS

PROS: Good internet coverage in urban areas and many islands, with reasonable pricing.

CONS: Internet service may be slower and less reliable in remote areas.

SAFETY

PROS: Greece is generally safe with low crime rates, especially in rural and island communities.

CONS: Petty crimes including pickpocketing can occur in busy tourist areas.

JUDICIAL

PROS: EU member with a structured legal system.

CONS: Legal processes can be slow; bureaucracy can be cumbersome for expats.

POLITICAL STABILITY

PROS: Greece has a stable political system within the EU framework.

CONS: Economic challenges and austerity measures have led to some social unrest and protests in the past. Primarily in cities.

CAMBODIA

Cambodia captivates visitors with its remarkable blend of enchanting history, hospitable culture, and affordability. This Southeast Asian nation is steeped in a rich past, evident in the majestic ruins of Angkor Wat and the vibrant tales woven through its cities and countryside.

The warmth of the Cambodian people, with their genuine smiles and open hearts, adds to the country's allure, making anyone feel at home. Coupled with the relatively low cost of living, Cambodia offers a compelling proposition for travelers and expatriates alike, seeking to immerse themselves in its unique heritage and laid-back lifestyle without straining their budgets.

CAPITAL: Phnom Penh

FOUR MAJOR CITIES: Phnom Penh, Siem Reap, Battambang, Sihanoukville

PRIMARY LANGUAGE: Khmer

CURRENCY: Cambodian Riel (KHR)

COUNTRY PHONE CODE: +855

MAJOR INDUSTRIES: Textiles, tourism, agriculture, construction

MAJOR EXPORTS: Clothing, rice, rubber, fish, tobacco

TYPE OF GOVERNMENT: Constitutional monarchy under a parliamentary democracy

RETIREE VISA: Cambodia offers specific visas for foreign retirees who can prove a stable source of income.

AVERAGE TEMPERATURE: Varies from 21°C to 35°C (70°F to 95°F) throughout the year

RELOCATION TO CAMBODIA: PROS AND CONS

Specific and Popular Places to Relocate to

PROS: Expatriates often choose Phnom Penh for its vibrant culture and Siem Reap for proximity to Angkor Wat. Coastal towns like Sihanoukville offer beautiful beaches, while Battambang presents a quieter, more authentic experience.

CONS: Popular areas can be crowded, with Siem Reap and Sihanoukville experiencing tourism peaks. Some may find Phnom Penh's rapid development and traffic overwhelming.

COST OF LIVING

PROS: Cambodia's low cost of living allows for a comfortable lifestyle on a modest budget, including dining out, accommodation, and transportation.

CONS: In major cities and tourist areas, prices can be significantly higher, especially for Western amenities and housing standards.

INFRASTRUCTURE

PROS: Urban areas, particularly Phnom Penh, are developing rapidly, with improving roads, healthcare facilities, and access to international goods.

CONS: Rural and remote areas may lack basic infrastructure, including reliable roads, making travel challenging.

UTILITIES

PROS: Eelectricity and water are generally affordable in urban areas.

CONS: Frequent power outages and inconsistent water supply can occur, especially outside major cities.

ACCESS TO AND COST OF HEALTHCARE

PROS: Affordable healthcare services and medications are available in major cities.

CONS: Quality of care varies significantly; serious medical issues often require travel to nearby countries like Thailand or Singapore.

CLIMATE

PROS: Warm, tropical climate year-round.

CONS: The hot, humid weather can be uncomfortable for some, and the monsoon season brings heavy rainfall.

FOOD

PROS: Delicious, diverse cuisine with a variety of local and international dishes at low prices.

CONS: Adjusting to local food hygiene standards can be challenging for newcomers.

ALCOHOL

PROS: Alcohol, particularly local beer, is very affordable.

CONS: The availability of quality imported alcohol can be limited and expensive.

SOCIAL LIFE

PROS: Vibrant expat communities and friendly locals make it easy to have an active social life.

CONS: Cultural and language barriers may hinder deeper connections with locals for some.

CULTURE

PROS: Rich cultural heritage with numerous festivals, traditions, and historical sites.

CONS: Adjusting to local norms and customs can take time for newcomers.

TRANSPORTATION

PROS: Affordable public transport options, including buses and tuk-tuks.

CONS: Traffic congestion in cities and safety standards for public transport can be concerning.

CAR HIRE AND FUEL

PROS: Car and motorbike rentals are readily available at reasonable rates.

CONS: Traffic conditions and driving habits can be challenging for foreigners, and fuel costs are relatively high.

INTERNET ACCESS

PROS: Good internet access in urban areas with reasonable monthly costs.

CONS: Internet reliability and speed can be inconsistent, particularly in rural areas.

SAFETY

PROS: Generally safe for expatriates and tourists, with low violent crime rates.

CONS: Petty theft and scams can be a concern, especially in tourist areas.

JUDICIAL

PROS: Legal processes for business and residency are straightforward for expatriates.

CONS: The legal system can be slow, and navigating it without local assistance can be complicated.

POLITICAL STABILITY

PROS: Cambodia has enjoyed relative political stability in recent years, encouraging economic growth and development.

CONS: Political rights and freedoms are limited, with occasional government crackdowns on dissent.

THE IMPORTANCE OF TRAVEL

I firmly believe that by setting new goals and embracing challenges, I will continue to invigorate my life as I age. Traveling ranks high among my personal favorite ways to do this, as even the shortest trip typically offers a plethora of fresh experiences that help to enrich my understanding of the world.

I find that the unique appeal of travel lies in how I am often serendipitously provided with input for all my senses. But travel is not just an eye-opening experience. I also often feel challenged both mentally and physically by experiencing new environments, trying foreign cuisines and engaging in new cultural activities. While this can at times be overwhelming, it's mostly immensely rewarding and helps to expand my worldview and deepen an appreciation of places that are unfamiliar and far from home.

Stepping out of my daily routine, even briefly, enhances my life. Since traveling usually promotes physical activity, whether it's exploring urban landscapes, hiking, or just casual beach walks, my physical and mental well-being also benefit.

Even short, spontaneous trips nearby my home can be enriching, offering new perspectives – without the need for extensive planning or expense. These local excursions are not only affordable but also provide a refreshing change of everyday, mundane pace.

That said, longer trips do tend to be more adventurous. Traveling to distant destinations brings about deeper, intense and therefore more lasting memories.

Extended journeys also offer more time for self-reflection, solitude, and learning, whether it's picking up new language skills, participating in local cultural events, or volunteering, thereby combining the joy of discovery with societal contribution.

In essence, traveling is more than just visiting new places; it's about rejuvenating life, embracing new knowledge, and investing in personal growth. Whether through a day trip, an extended adventure or a residential relocation, the transformative power of stepping out of our comfort zone, challenging as it can be at times, is always rewarding.

In this chapter, we've explored some of the considerations that should be part of a robust retirement plan – ranging from financial strategies and healthcare to lifestyle preferences and housing options.

My goal has been to provide you with a clearer picture of the practical steps needed to secure a comfortable future, as well as to spark ideas about how you might enrich your life with new experiences, whether through relocation or by simply redefining your day-to-day activities.

As you move forward, remember that retirement isn't just about managing finances or maintaining health, though these are undeniably important variables. It's also about seizing the opportunity to fulfill long-held dreams and explore new passions.

Ultimately, this chapter should serve as a launchpad for you to begin planning, encourage thinking about your future, and inspire you to perhaps take bold steps toward designing a retirement that echoes your personal aspirations and ideals. This isn't just about ending a career; it's about beginning perhaps the most personally rewarding chapter of your life.

CHAPTER 10

The Aging Man's Survival Guide

BRIGHTER DAYS AHEAD

How embracing a positive
perspective promotes health.

I've dedicated this chapter to the surprisingly powerful impact that adopting a positive mindset can have on us as we navigate the sometimes gnarly male aging process. It focuses on how locating silver linings and reframing challenges as opportunities for growth can make this part of life considerably more enjoyable and interesting!

I'll also share how embracing positivity can boost mental health, strengthen social ties and help us overcome feelings of irrelevancy and isolation as we grow older.

THE POWER OF POSITIVITY

At 60, I am at the beginning of what is arguably the most transformative period of my adult life. As with most men, the pace and particulars of my aging process are and will continue to be influenced by genetic, environmental, and lifestyle variables. So far, I've experienced it as being both a rather slow and subtle process but certainly with episodes of more rapid and seismic change.

One aspect of the aging process that is in fact within our immediate control is attitude, mindset, and how we choose to face the aging process.

By consciously cultivating a positive outlook and embracing instead of rejecting or even denying, the shifts that come with getting older, we can profoundly impact most experiences and actually improve the quality of life.

Although exactly how we perceive our senior years can vary greatly from person to person, the effects of aging will touch on most aspects of life, including our health, our relationships, and for some, even impact us financially.

For me, embracing positivity has proven to be a very powerful and lasting way to help smooth over some of the unavoidable trials and tribulations that have come my way during the aging process.

At the very least, I've found that maintaining an optimistic attitude has significantly softened the psychological jolts when tougher challenges every so often surprise and even overwhelm me.

Just by simply being more aware – mindful – that there will be struggles and that I will eventually overcome them and, if necessary, adapt, has helped strengthen my confidence and emotional stability.

I've also realized how both body and mind are connected to my overall well-being and long-term health, much more so than fleeting pleasures and the escapism I enjoy from occasional indulgences.

SMILING

As I've aged, I've noticed the impact gravity has had on, among other places, my face. Though not necessarily a reflection of my mood or attitude, today's default resting expression tends to look less cheerful and optimistic.

After acknowledging this, I've used the realization as a reminder to smile more often for the positive effect smiling literally has on how I look and how I am perceived. But I also smile to see if it can have an impact on others.

Smiling has become a conscious way for me to counteract the physical signs of aging and remind myself and others that I am still a mostly happy and approachable fellow.

CONTAGIOUS OPTIMISM

We tend to gravitate towards people who radiate happiness and optimism. This is likely because positivity is contagious; it uplifts the mood of others and makes most social exchanges, if not always enjoyable, then at least less frictional..

I don't always feel positive and refuse to act like I am. But whenever I'm able find a way to have a more positive perspective, the "rewards" I receive are always detectable. Being a beacon of positivity seems to invite more worthwhile and purposeful social interactions in my life.

MENTAL HEALTH

Understanding the mental health benefits of positivity does not necessitate a degree in Behavioral Psychology. I know for a fact that when I embrace a positive perspective as opposed to one characterized by pessimism and negativism, I can more easily compartmentalize or dilute problems and challenges.

While this method doesn't immediately solve anything, it definitely reduces stress and the risk of letting problems get me down and making me feel gloomy. Turns out that given some perspective and time, most daily obstacles and difficulties can usually be solved with just a little elbow grease. Or, better yet, by reframing them.

CREATIVITY AND PROBLEM-SOLVING

Over the years, having a positive attitude has been key in increasing my creative thinking and problem-solving abilities. Whenever I encounter challenges, I try to see where the opportunities are rather than just take inventory of the observable problems, which leads me to discover interesting solutions and novel ways to effectively resolve them.

Being optimistic also boosts my productivity as it instills in me a sense of confidence, motivates me to take action and not put off challenges. It's the compass that guides me toward successful outcomes, especially when I face hurdles and setbacks.

In my mind, there's no doubt that positivity is crucial in developing resilience – the ability to recover from bad luck, poor judgment or a combination of both. In challenging times, a positive attitude allows me to be more effective at coping which in turn helps facilitate quicker recovery and provides valuable learning from my experiences. Good and bad.

MINDFULNESS AND POSITIVITY

Integrating mindfulness practices like Yoga, Qigong, meditation and deep breathing exercises, often helps me return to positive thinking. These and other exercises allow me to stay focused on the present and appreciate the current moment as well as reduce the clutter and chatter of negative thoughts.

MAINTAINING A POSITIVE MINDSET

Despite numerous benefits, I'm the first to admit that maintaining a positive attitude can often be tough, especially during a string of mishaps and periods of extreme stress. Life's trials can evoke strong negative emotions, and I think it's important to not always try to deny or suppress these feelings.

I think setting realistic expectations is important. Positivity is not about perpetual happiness or avoiding life's difficulties; it's about sustaining hope and finding joy or learning lessons even while dealing with tough circumstances. For me, acknowledging problems and processing negative emotions – in a healthy way – is the key to returning to positivity.

POSITIVE ENVIRONMENT

In a world where negative headlines and soundbites are ever-present – and where a big part of the news media's business model is to sensationalize journalism in order to attract as many viewers and readers as possible, it can be testing to always keep a positive attitude and perspective.

Surrounding ourselves with positive influences, be it is through the choice of people we listen to, socialize with, the information we choose to engage with, or the activities we opt to commit to, that can help reinforce our optimistic outlook. Making a conscious effort and being consistent are also important ingredients in maintaining a positive approach to the challenges of daily life.

REFRAMING

The idea that there is always a brighter way to view a problem or obstacle in life is the very concept of positive reframing. It suggests that by identifying and concentrating on the positive characteristics of even a troublesome situation, we can more effectively overcome hurdles, navigate hardships, and liberate ourselves from the bonds of negativity and pessimism.

It's not just about blind optimism; it involves a strategic and mindful shift in perspective that can lead to real, tangible benefits.

UNDERSTANDING POSITIVE REFRAMING

PERSPECTIVE SHIFT

Positive reframing is about shifting our perspective in order to focus on the silver lining in any given dire circumstance.

In my life, in order to find the silver lining in particularly rough situations, I've had to look at things in a totally different way to see beyond the immediate pain and consider the potential for positive angles that are inherit to everything from small problems to stupendous adversities.

RELATIONSHIPS

In younger years, the end of a relationship could often be heart-wrenching. Yet, in the aftermath, I could have a period of self-discovery and personal growth. Eventually, the void the broken relationship forced me to evolve and engage in new and more compatible relationships.

FINANCIAL

In my career, whenever freelance work was scarce and I was having trouble meeting financial goals and responsibilities, the stress and uncertainty could be almost debilitating. But these unexpected pauses allowed me to reassess my goals and learn new skills that I might never have explored otherwise and would prove to make me more relevant.

Experiencing financial hardship taught me invaluable lessons about budgeting, the importance of having financial foresight and planning for periods with less work. It also encouraged me to accept a simpler lifestyle and find happiness in having less things. Most importantly, is strengthened my resolve to never give up.

HEALTH

Facing illness related to getting older has also brought its own set of challenges, testing my resilience in ways I never imagined I would have to endure when I was younger.

My physical ailments also deepened my appreciation for life and motivated me to commit to a healthier lifestyle. It was a difficult time, but it also brought our family closer and inspired those around us.

AGING

I've enjoyed jogging for most of my adult life. But I'm also an avid walker and enjoy taking long strolls regularly, especially when traveling and where I don't have access to a gym or a good place to run.

I've recently noticed that my walking speed has slowed down a bit. While some might see this as a limitation, I've reframed this and can now see it as an opportunity to enjoy more of everything that surrounds me. My new slower tempo also provides me with a great opportunity to listen more to audiobooks and podcasts.

SEX

Similarly, while the frequency of sexual intimacy has become less with age, I've discovered that the intensity has increased substantially whenever it does happen, making each occasion imbued with a newfound depth of emotion and pleasure that was perhaps overlooked in the rush of my younger years. It's a reminder that quality often trumps quantity.

RETAINING RELEVANCE

And as for relevance, which I've covered at some length in the chapter Staying Relevant, it's certainly true that the professional world no longer sees me in the same light as it once did. Fortunately, as a life-long creative and curious individual, I have encouraged myself to explore and pursue new ways to help redefine my identity and relevancy – professionally and socially.

Whether by traveling to new places, meeting new people or exposing myself to new knowledge, I've found that relevance is not lost at all. It has simply evolved. It's all about adapting and being open the opportunities that change can give life to.

My journey of aging, with all its physical, emotional and psychological transitions, has taught me that there's always a silver lining and a way to reframe any given situation – if I'm only willing to embrace a positive perspective and an optimistic attitude.

Through each of these experiences, I've learned that difficulties are not just hurdles to overcome; they can also be an invitation to grow, to redefine life, and to find strength and happiness in places I hadn't even thought to look.

COGNITIVE FLEXIBILITY

This is a process that requires a flexible mindset – the ability to think about situations in multiple ways and fluidly adapt to new information as it flows in. "Zooming out" from almost any difficult situation can make looking at it objectively easier. Not just seeing it from a single, subjective, often emotionally charged perspective.

Shining light on a problem from an entirely different angle can provide an unexpected opportunity to discover a new solution. It's not about denying the difficulty of a situation per se, rather acknowledging the challenge while also recognizing the opportunities, the silver lining it presents.

Adopting this mindset has prompted me to look for creative solutions and hone my problem-solving skills rather than just contemplate or, worse, procrastinate. By focusing on how to figure out a means to overcome an issue, I also feel like I'm cognitively better equipped to handle future problems.

Again, this approach does not negate the reality of hardships but instead provides a balanced perspective that emphasizes resilience and the potential for growth. By practicing being positive in a realistic way, we can develop a more robust and adaptable mindset, enabling us to more easily leap over hurdles, tunnel our way through austerity, and break free from the chains of negativity.

I realize that it's not a one-size-fits-all solution, but rather a very personalized one that varies from one individual to another. It involves a consistent, ongoing process of self-reflection and adjustment to a more flexible and fluid thought pattern and attitude.

The key lies in recognizing the power of perspective and consciously choosing to focus on the aspects of any situation that can lead to a positive outcome.

Incorporating this into daily life can start with small steps – like simply acknowledging small victories in a difficult day. Over time, this shift in perspective can transform how challenges are perceived, leading to a more optimistic, positive life experience.

Ultimately, the practice of focusing on positives in the face of life's inescapable challenges is a testament to the human spirit's ability and capacity to withstand, learn and adjust.

I see this is a solid reminder that even in the darkest of times, there is always some light to be found. And by focusing on this light, we empower ourselves to move forward with strength and positivity.

AVOIDING TOXIC POSITIVITY

There's a fine line between positive reframing and toxic positivity – the latter being an overgeneralization of a positive outlook that ignores and or dismisses real issues that need to be addressed. Pretending everything is okay when it's not, can lead to invalidating genuine problems that demand focus to be solved.

While it's beneficial to always try and see things in a positive light, to locate the silver lining, it can become really harmful when this perspective stops us from acknowledging and dealing with real-life problems we face.

MANTRAS FOR POSITIVITY

Here are a few of my personal mantras that help remind me of being positive and keeping an optimistic mindset. Repeating one or several of these mantras daily can help instill a more supportive outlook, transform thought patterns, and increase an overall sense of well-being.

I am enough just as I am.

I embrace the ebb and flow of my life

Secretly, my challenges help me.

Every day is a fresh start with plenty of Easter eggs (hidden gems).

I am strong and brave.

I have more faith than doubt.

I trust the journey, even when I do not understand it.

I thrive on positive and healthy relationships.

I am constantly evolving.

My smile radiates positivity.

My heart is open to love and joy.

I choose to find the good in every situation.

I am at peace with my past and excited about my future.

I have the power to create change in my life.

I am guided by hope, and courage.

Dealing with "Drainers"

The older I get, the more my tolerance for negativity and pessimism dwindles. Now more than ever, I find immense value in surrounding myself with individuals who radiate, creativity, positivity and optimism.

This conscious choice to engage with friends and family who uplift and inspire me has become an important part of my approach to life as an aging man.

As previously discussed in this chapter, the infectious nature of positivity can significantly enhance our outlook on life. In the same vein, a negative mindset can spread with equal ease, burdening me with additional stress atop existing issues that I am in various stages of dealing with.

Choosing positivity is not just about seeking joy but also about actively deciding to lighten the load of aging's challenges. By aligning myself with those who embody hope and happiness, I feel I am better equipped to navigate life with confidence and gratitude, and make each moment of my life count.

The concept of "Drainers" refers to individuals characterized by a persistently negative outlook on life in general and everything bad that happens to them. They are the eternal victims.

These people often view situations pessimistically, embodying the 'glass half empty' mentality and are likely to subscribe to conspiracy theories that prove how their own misfortune and shortcomings stem from the ill will of others and are not their fault – or their responsibility!

Drainers are not confined to any specific group; they can be found among friends, family members, acquaintances, or colleagues. Their defining trait is an ability to deplete the positive energy of those around them, often leaving people feeling emotionally drained and exhausted.

CHARACTERISTICS OF DRAINERS

A PESSIMISTIC WORLDVIEW

Some drainers view life through a lens of negativity. They focus on problems rather than solutions and often expect the worst outcomes.

EMOTIONAL VAMPIRISM

Drainers seem to feed off the positive energy of others, often monopolizing conversations with their troubles and worries, leaving little room for positive or constructive dialogue.

CHRONIC COMPLAINERS

Drainers often incessantly complain about various aspects of their lives, work, relationships, or society without actively seeking solutions. They tend to resist change or taking advice despite their constant grievances and prefer to remain in their negative mindset.

IMPACT ON OTHERS

Regular interactions with a Drainer can leave you feeling emotionally depleted and you may even find yourself becoming more pessimistic and negative after spending time with them.

LACK OF RECIPROCITY

Relationships with Drainers often feel one-sided, with your efforts to support or uplift them going unreciprocated. This might encourage you to start dreading interactions with them, anticipating the emotional toll it usually takes.

SETTING BOUNDARIES WITH DRAINERS

I've tried to establish clear boundaries with the few Drainers I still have a relationship with in order to protect my emotional well-being. From time to time I offer constructive feedback that firmly communicates how their negativity impacts me. Still, since Drainers are typically so full of themselves and usually unaware of their effect on me, I am steadily limiting my exposure to them.

UNDERLYING ISSUES

Often, Drainers' negativity stems from unresolved personal issues, including low self-esteem, past traumas, or chronic stress. They might lack effective coping mechanisms to deal with life's challenges, resorting to negativity as a defense mechanism.

Sometimes, their behavior is a way to seek attention or sympathy from others. For some Drainers, negativity has become a habitual response to life, deeply ingrained in their personality.

By setting boundaries, maintaining a positive environment, and focusing on your own emotional health, you can effectively manage these challenging relationships while preserving your own positivity and peace of mind.

BRIGHTER DAYS ARE AHEAD

As I reflect on my life now as a man passed the milestone of 60, growing older has certainly brought its own set of challenges. Some mornings, I wake with aches in places I didn't know could ache. Other days, memories seem a little less sharp than yesterday.

Yet, despite knowing that these changes are natural, it's taking some time to accept what I now know is a profound truth: by maintaining a positive perspective, I can illuminate days when it might otherwise get pretty dark. Looking forward, not back, has become my mantra. In my younger days, like many men, it was easy to be consumed by past accomplishments and achieved goals. I had a career that many would call successful, and yes, there were times when I perhaps leaned a bit too heavily on past achievements and could be both self-congratulatory and boastful.

But what I've come to realize is that dwelling on past glories can cast a long shadow on the present, and even limit new opportunities in my social life.

Generally speaking, people aren't drawn to us solely because of what we've done; they're attracted to who we are now and what we still want to achieve. I've learned that acting self-important can be isolating, pushing away the very connections that we crave and need as we grow older.

We all have stories to tell, but what makes life interesting now, at least for me, is sharing new experiences with others and creating new stories together.

By adopting an open and humble attitude towards life's possibilities, I've opened doors I never knew were there. It's about being honest about where I am today, not just where I've been.

By showing genuine interest in others and being honest about both successes and failures, I've made myself open to new relationships and strengthened old ones. This openness has not only kept me relevant but has also allowed me to grow and inspire other.

Each day offers a new beginning, a new chance to reframe challenges into opportunities. Whether it's learning a new skill, exploring unfamiliar places, or simply taking the time to listen and learn from others, every moment is a chance to shine light into what might initially seem like darkness.

In this part of life, I am convinced that brighter days lie not behind me, but ahead of me. It's all about perspective. Embracing the present and looking forward to the future with optimism and humility doesn't just help navigate the aging process – it literally transforms it into a journey that continues to be as fulfilling as it is surprising.

The next chapter, Improving & Extending Life will offer even more ideas and advice on this topic.

CHAPTER 11

The Aging Man's Survival Guide

STAYING RELEVANT

Evolving, adapting and thriving with age.

There are many ways to maintain relevance – especially after our professional life has come to an end. This chapter includes thoughts and ideas about the importance of socializing, networking, mentorship, volunteering, and how even becoming a pet owner can significantly help create a new kind of social relevance.

As we age, our role in society, among friends, and within our family should continue to thrive and play an important part of our identity. Proactively maintaining our relevance as we grow older can therefore be a stimulating and a health-promoting goal well worth pursuing with both enthusiasm and determination.

Of course, this requires a combination of willingness to adapt to new circumstances, and a commitment to keep meaningful social connections going and perhaps leave destructive relationships behind.

AVOIDING LONELINESS

Sadly, I've noticed a troubling trend, not just in my own life but in the lives of many of my peers: isolation and loneliness. For some, the social fabric that once held life together begins to fray once retirement sets in.

Retirement, but also the loss of loved ones, and physical limitations can drastically shrink our world. I've seen friends and family members retreat into shells of their former selves, often feeling unwanted or forgotten. This isolation isn't just sad; it's also detrimental to their health – mentally, physically, and emotionally.

Mentally, isolation clouds our thinking and can lead to depression. Physically, studies have shown that loneliness can increase the risk of conditions like heart disease. Emotionally, the despair of feeling disconnected from the world can erode our sense of purpose and induce an existential crisis.

The easiest way to combat loneliness is by maintaining our relevance. Staying connected with the world isn't just about social engagements – it's also about feeling needed and valued. By sharing our life experiences and wisdom with friends and family, especially with younger generations, we can maintain a sense of purpose.

Staying relevant helps avoid the pitfalls of loneliness by keeping us engaged in a world that appreciates our participation and values our presence. It reminds us that no matter our age, we have something to offer.

There are many ways to maintain and increase relevance. Here are some simple yet hopefully inspiring ideas and why I think they can help.

STAY CURIOUS

Committing to curiosity by trying out new hobbies and learning new skills – especially if they seem to stretch our mental capacity or exceed our physical boundaries, or both – can help reconfigure our identity and increase our relevance as we grow older.

Engagement in learning can take a myriad of forms and include academic level education, mastering a new practical skill that demands both discipline and creativity, opening a window to a completely new culture and learning a new language.

Even the relatively simple act of reading or listening to podcasts or audio books about unfamiliar subjects can spark curiosity and lead to insights about the world and our place within it.

For me, podcasts usually serve as an inspiring gateway to new ideas that often challenge both ignorance and preconceived notions.

Having a commitment to learning and growing, to embracing the unknown and the unfamiliar, cultivates a mindset that flourishes from exploration and discovery. It encourages us to remain open and adaptable which are qualities that can even seem to slow down our aging process.

STAY TECHNOLOGICALLY FIT

In today's era of ever-evolving digital communication, I think it's important to stay reasonably up-to-date with technology. For example, as addictive and at times toxic as it can be, many social media platforms can still offer significant value since they allow us to stay connected, in real-time, with friends, family, current and former colleagues, regardless of time or geographical distances.

By scheduling specific times of day for checking social media and adhering to these time slots – whether it's a half-hour in the morning and evening or short checks after lunch, can help us keep a balanced usage and avoid risks of overuse.

Turning off non-essential notifications to avoid being drawn into unplanned social media use can also help maintain control over digital engagement and keep the limited social media schedule intact.

I try to approach social media with clear intentions. I identify what I want to achieve – be it staying in touch with family, following news, or participating in specific interest groups –and focus my activity accordingly.

Having a healthy embrace of technology and learning to use new digital tools to keep up with the changing world can help us from feeling left behind. But it's important to be mindful about when it's time to take a break and perhaps just pick up a phone and call, or, maybe even write a letter!

MENTORSHIP

Becoming a mentor allows us to share our knowledge and experience accumulated over time and contribute to the growth and development of those we help.

The act of mentorship not only helps others learn and advance in their careers or personal lives, it also provides us with a way to maintain relevance in our own, including at former workplaces, in our neighborhood, and community.

By offering guidance, advice, and support in the capacity of a mentor or personal advisor, we can also stay connected and learn both evolving trends and totally new things, which makes sure that our skills and insights remain valuable and up-to-date.

NETWORKING

Now that I am over 60, actively avoiding isolation has become important for my mental and emotional well-being.

It's no secret that isolation can lead to feelings of loneliness, depression, and a decline in physical health, which makes it essential to actively engage in social activities and be open to expanding my social circle.

By exposing ourselves to opportunities where we meet new people and possibly forge new friendships, we can experience a renewed sense of belonging and purpose. Engaging with others, whether through shared hobbies, volunteer work, or community events, inevitably stimulates our mind, and can strengthen us emotionally.

The gist is this, whether you feel it or not, most social interactions, even the most mundane, can actually improve our lives. Maintaining an active social life is therefore not just about filling time; it's about securing the quality of life and experiencing the profound fulfillment that comes from social connections and from being open to entirely new acquaintances and potentially, long-lasting friendships.

EMBRACE CHANGE

In my experience, being flexible to change and willing to adapt to new circumstances is not just good for me mentally; it also improves my social vitality. The world is in a constant state of flux, and the ability to pivot, adjust, and evolve is important for maintaining my relevance socially. Adaptability invites a more flexible mindset, enabling me to navigate the uncertainties this stage of life throws at me with more elasticity and confidence.

By being open to change, we are encouraging a learning attitude, making sure that we remain mentally sharp and emotionally strong.

Taking on new challenges, learning new skills, adopting technologies, or even embracing new cultural trends can significantly improve the quality of life and open up opportunities for new experiences and social connections.

It's about not letting age define our capabilities but rather use the insights that come with experience and wisdom to approach change with confidence and unapologetic enthusiasm.

POSITIVE RELATIONSHIPS

I try hard to stay involved in the lives of family and friends by attending family gatherings and making an effort to reach out to old friends. This helps me maintain my emotional stability and well-being. Strong personal relationships often act as a foundation for happiness and support, offering both comfort and companionship.

It's also important to consider nurturing relationships with former colleagues and business contacts, even post-retirement. These connections can enrich life by providing a sense of connection to one's history.

Social networking, regardless of age, opens doors to new and exciting opportunities, encouraging a vibrant social life filled with meaningful social interactions and personal growth.

By actively maintaining these relationships, we can ensure a network of support and engagement that benefits both mental and emotional health.

END DESTRUCTIVE RELATIONSHIPS

In my experience, destructive relationships are often characterized by chronic conflicts, emotional abuse, repetitive manipulation, and overall negativity. Scientific research has documented how unhealthy dynamics in a relationship inevitably lead to elevated levels of the stress-induced hormone cortisol.

Prolonged exposure to high levels of cortisol is associated with a range of health problems, including high blood pressure, impaired immune function, cardiovascular issues, and cognitive decline. The fact is, our ability to manage stress can become compromised, making us more vulnerable to its negative effects the older we get.

In addition to these physical health risks, the emotional toll of destructive relationships usually cause a lot of anxiety and sometimes severe depression as well as a diminished sense of self-worth. So, it's crucial to recognize the signs of a destructive relationship and take steps to either improve the relationship or, if necessary, disengage from it altogether.

BE SUPPORTIVE

Offering support and guidance to the younger members of your family is not only a generous and fulfilling act but also a vital part of family dynamics.

As an older family member, you possess a wealth of experiences and wisdom gained from your journey through life's challenges and ups and downs.

Our accumulated knowledge can be an invaluable resource and help a younger generation navigate the uncertainties of their own lives.

Sharing personal experiences, both the successes and the lessons learned from mistakes, can provide family members with a roadmap to make more informed decisions.

Guidance can cover a wide range of topics, from career choices and financial planning to matters of the heart and personal development. By sharing insights, we can help those younger than us avoid common pitfalls and inspire them to explore their full potential.

A willingness to offer support can be a source of comfort, reminding them that they have a safety net within the family when facing difficulties. It also strengthens the bonds between generations, reinforcing the idea that a family is a place of trust, mentorship, and unconditional love.

Your wisdom serves as a bridge between generations, ensuring that valuable life lessons are passed down and preserved, enriching the family's collective understanding and nurturing the growth of its youngest members.

VOLUNTEERING & COMMUNITY INVOLVEMENT

Volunteer work, whether within in our own community or by traveling abroad, offers a uniquely enriching experience that extends beyond mere personal growth. It's a chance to connect with a new cultures in a new environment, and with new individuals, all while making a tangible difference.

Volunteering allows us to step outside our daily routine and contribute to causes that need immediate attention, from environmental conservation to education and healthcare.

An altruistic journey can broaden perspectives and provide a sense of global citizenship and empathy. It can also provide invaluable skills, experiences, and memories that enrich life profoundly.

By choosing to volunteer, you're not just helping others; you're embarking on an adventure that will likely transform your understanding of the world and place within it, fill life with purpose, joy, and the satisfaction that comes from knowing you've made an important contribution.

HERE ARE A FEW IDEAS OF HOW TO GET INVOLVED IN VOLUNTEERING

TUTORING AND TEACHING

Local schools and educational programs often welcome volunteers who can tutor or teach students. With a wealth of life experience and knowledge, you can provide guidance and support students.

Whether it's helping with homework, career insights, or sharing your love for reading, writing, or solving math problems, this role can have a profound impact on a student's appreciation for academics and inspire his or her educational journey tremendously.

SENIOR COMPANIONSHIP

Volunteering at senior centers, assisted living facilities, nursing homes, or retirement communities can provide a unique opportunity to make a tangible difference in the lives of older adults.

This kind of community service can offer you unique personal connections by for example, participating in shared activities, or just by lending an empathetic ear to those who might often feel overlooked or undervalued.

For many older adults, the interactions you can provide will certainly enhance their quality of life by adding social stimulation, and a sense of belonging.

For you, as the volunteer, the experience can be equally rewarding, as it can offer a sense of fulfillment and purpose, knowing you have contributed positively to someone's day-to-day well-being. Engaging in volunteer work not only bridges generational gaps but also promotes a culture of care and respect, reinforcing the value of every individual at any stage of life.

ENVIRONMENTAL STEWARDSHIP

I highly recommend getting involved in local conservation efforts, like participating in clean-up projects at public beaches or planting trees in community parks. These activities not only contribute to the enhancement of our local environment but also offer a profound sense of personal achievement and fulfillment.

This kind of volunteer work can provide a fantastic opportunity for you to stay physically active and enjoy the beauty of the outdoors. It can also contribute a sense of community and shared purpose among all participants, uniting them in the commitment to ecological stewardship.

By taking part, you'll not only be improving your own physical health but also connecting with like-minded individuals. Together, you'll be part of a dedicated network of environmental advocates, making a difference in your community and sending a clear message to others that what you do matters.

COMMUNITY ORGANIZING

Historically, community organizing has played a pivotal role in bringing about social change and improvement at the local level. Across various communities, grassroots organizations work tirelessly on a wide range of issues, including housing, healthcare, and poverty alleviation, aiming to create a more equitable and supportive society.

By getting involved, you too can have the opportunity to contribute meaningfully to addressing some of the most pressing needs within your neighborhood and community. Participation can take various forms, from advocacy and raising awareness about specific issues to organizing fundraising campaigns that provide vital resources for community projects.

Engaging in these activities not only helps to bring about tangible changes but also strengthens the community's collective voice, making it possible to achieve significant impact.

Involvement in grassroots initiatives can also offer a unique chance to develop a deeper understanding of the challenges facing your community, advancing empathy and solidarity among members.

CRISIS SUPPORT AND DISASTER RELIEF

Volunteering with charitable organizations and NGOs and local disaster relief agencies, offers an invaluable avenue to provide critical support in times of crisis. When emergencies occur, be it natural disasters or human-made calamities, the immediate assistance volunteers provide can be life-saving.

Roles in disaster response are diverse, ranging from on-the-ground efforts like delivering first aid and emergency medical services to logistical support like coordinating shelter and distributing essential supplies to affected individuals and families.

This type of volunteer work not only demands courage and a willingness to help under pressure but can also provide you with a profound sense of fulfillment from making a tangible difference in the lives of those caught in the midst of devastating situations. By stepping into this volunteer role, you become a crucial pillar of resilience and recovery, helping others navigate the challenging aftermath of a disaster.

HEALTHCARE VOLUNTEERING

Hospitals and healthcare facilities frequently rely on the generosity of volunteers to enhance their capacity to care for patients and support their families.

By assisting with various tasks like transporting patients between departments, offering comfort and reassurance to families waiting on news of their loved ones, or running errands for patients who have no one else to turn to, you can play a critical role in enhancing the healthcare environment.

This type of volunteering not only alleviates some of the operational pressures on medical staff, allowing them to focus more on patient care, but also directly impacts the well-being of patients and their families by providing a more compassionate and supportive environment.

Engaging in volunteer work offers a unique opportunity to contribute positively to the community, witness the direct results of kindness and understand the profound difference a simple act of goodwill can make in the lives of people going through challenging times.

LIBRARY AND MUSEUM ASSISTANCE

If you have an appreciation for literature, art, or history, volunteering at a local library or museum could be a great opportunity to combine your interest and contribute to the community.

Many culturally-focused institutions rely on the support of volunteers to run a wide array of activities, from organizing events and leading tours to assisting with educational programs that enrich the community's knowledge and appreciation of cultural heritage.

This role can allow you to immerse yourself in your passions and also provide a platform to share that enthusiasm with others, potentially inspiring the same love for learning and culture in them.

It's a fulfilling way to ensure that libraries and museums remain vibrant centers of education and cultural exploration. Plus, it offers the personal benefit of meeting others who share your interests, allowing for the exchange of ideas and fostering a sense of connection and belonging within your local cultural scene.

HOME REPAIR AND MAINTENANCE

Another meaningful way to contribute to your community is volunteering with organizations that provide free home repair and maintenance services to those in need, including low-income families and the elderly. Your time and effort can help ensure that those most in need have a safe and comfortable place to call home.

These organizations welcome volunteers of all skill levels, from those with experience in various trades to others just eager to learn and then lend a hand. Getting involved in making crucial repairs and improvements to homes that are at risk of falling into disrepair, from fixing leaky roofs and reinforcing structures to ensuring that heating and plumbing are in working order, can directly improve the living conditions and safety of vulnerable community members.

By giving your time to these causes, you're also helping to lift the financial strain off individuals who can't afford necessary home repairs on their own. Your support can make a huge difference, offering everyone, regardless of their economic status or age, a chance to live in a secure and dignified environment. It's a rewarding opportunity to make a tangible impact and connect with others who share a commitment to making the community a better place for everyone.

MEAL DELIVERY AND FOOD BANKS

For a truly impactful way to give back to your community, consider volunteering at a local food bank or participating in meal delivery services for homebound individuals. This type of volunteer work is an important way of combating hunger and plays a critical role in making sure that those who are most vulnerable among us have access to the essential nourishment they need.

It's not just about the act of providing food; it's about offering hope and a touch of human kindness to those who might be facing difficult times. The gratitude you receive from those you help, and the knowledge that you're making a tangible difference in their lives, can be very fulfilling. Plus, it's a great way to connect with like-minded people who share your inclination to make a positive impact. Whether it's sorting and packaging meals at the food bank or delivering them, your contribution will be a beacon of support in your community.

ANIMAL SHELTER VOLUNTEERING

Volunteering at an animal shelter can not only be a deeply rewarding and heartwarming experience but also offer several of benefits that extend far beyond just filling spare time. It presents an excellent opportunity to stay physically and socially active, fostering a sense of purpose and relevance.

Engaging in tasks such as walking dogs, socializing with cats, maintaining kennels, or assisting with adoptions, volunteers provide essential care and support to animals waiting for their forever homes.

In addition to potentially reducing feelings of loneliness, depression, and anxiety, it also fosters a strong sense of responsibility and compassion towards animals in need.

The unconditional love and companionship these animals offer can become a surprisingly important part of one's life, making volunteering at an animal shelter an opportunity to be a voice for those who cannot speak for themselves.

The bonds formed with the animals and the satisfaction of helping them find loving families contribute to a deeply fulfilling volunteer experience, offering profound emotional and social rewards.

PET OWNERSHIP

Owning a pet, especially a dog or cat, can dramatically enhance social connections, reduce stress levels, and lead to a more fulfilling life.

The bond with a pet not only encourages physical activity but can also have a positive impact on mental health by lifting mood, bolstering self-esteem, and instilling a sense of purpose.

The companionship of a pet provides consistent interaction and affection, both of which are vital for emotional well-being and can significantly mitigate feelings of loneliness.

The presence of a pet can fill a home with life and energy and make it feel less empty and solitary. For many, especially those who live alone or are older, pets are often seen as a friend, offering unconditional love and comfort which can reduce the sense of isolation that can sometimes pervade life as we age.

It's important to keep in mind that pet ownership also comes with responsibilities including feeding, exercise, and social interaction. Having a pet can also pose challenges on your daily routines, spontaneous activities and your ability to travel.

Nonetheless, the key to fully enjoying pet ownership lies in finding a balance between these demands and the immense emotional and social rewards having a pet in your life brings.

The social aspect of owning a pet offers significant benefits, helping to create connections with other pet owners and even reduce feelings of loneliness.

Dog owners, for example, often engage in social interactions during walks in dog parks or visits to other dog-friendly venues, which can lead to meaningful relationships with fellow dog enthusiasts.

Similarly, cat owners typically connect with a community of cat lovers online and at cat cafes where they can share experiences and advice.

The companionship of a pet does more than just improve the bond between animal and human; it fosters important human connections, enriching the social lives of owners.

CHOOSING THE RIGHT PET

When deciding to buy a dog or cat, several important considerations will ensure you choose a pet that matches your lifestyle, expectations and ability to make a long-term commitment. Owning a dog or a cat is a significant decision that impacts not just your life but the well-being of the animal. Taking the following into account before making your choice will help ensure a harmonious match that brings joy to both you and your new pal.

PET SIZE

The size of a dog can significantly influence your living situation. Larger dogs typically need more space and may not be ideal for small apartments.

LIFE EXPECTANCY

Different breeds have varying life spans. Some dog breeds, like smaller ones, tend to live longer than larger breeds. Cats, especially mixed breeds, can often live into their late teens or early twenties with proper care.

FUR SHEDDING

Consider whether you're prepared to deal with shedding. Some dog and cat breeds shed very little, making them suitable for people with allergies or those who prefer not to deal with constant fur cleanup.

EXERCISE NEEDS

The amount of exercise a pet requires can vary dramatically between breeds. High-energy dog breeds like Border Collies or Jack Russell Terriers need more physical activity than more sedentary breeds.

Cats generally require less structured exercise but benefit from play that stimulates their hunting instincts.

SUSCEPTIBILITY TO DISEASES

Some pet breeds are more prone to certain genetic diseases than others. Researching the common health issues associated with your preferred breed can help you prepare for or possibly prevent these conditions. Here you might also want to consider healthcare and insurance costs.

TRAINABILITY

The ease with which a dog can learn commands and adapt to training varies among breeds. Some, like Golden Retrievers and Poodles, are known for their intelligence and trainability, while others may require more patience and effort.

FOOD CONSUMPTION

Larger pets typically consume more food, which can impact your budget. The dietary needs of your pet will depend on their size, age, and energy level, so consider this recurring expense.

TRAVELABILITY

Your ability to take your pet on public transportation can depend on the pet's size and the travel carrier you have. Smaller pets are generally easier to travel with, but even large dog breeds can be accommodated on many forms of transportation – with the right planning.

PASSION PURSUITS

As we age, it becomes increasingly important to challenge the brain in new and varied ways. Our daily routines, while comfortably familiar, can lead to a certain level of cognitive predictability.

This predictability, in turn, may not provide the mental stimulation necessary to keep our cognitive functions firing on all cylinders. The introduction of new hobbies can act as a catalyst for neuroplasticity, the brain's remarkable ability to form new neural connections – regardless of age.

This process of engaging in new passions not only revitalizes the brain but also contributes significantly to our emotional health. For instance, learning to play a musical instrument or picking up a new language not only demands cognitive effort – which in itself is beneficial – but also instills a sense of achievement and satisfaction.

The psychological benefits of overcoming challenges and learning new skills cannot be overstated; they imbue us with a renewed sense of purpose and invigorate our zest for life.

New activities also provide a platform for social interaction, which is a crucial element in maintaining mental health and emotional well-being. Joining clubs or groups that share new hobby can open up opportunities to meet like-minded people and invite social connections that might not have been possible otherwise.

Social interactions can be particularly enriching by offering emotional support, enhancing our sense of belonging, and even reducing feelings of loneliness or isolation.

The pursuit of new hobbies also serves as a stress reliever, offering a much-needed break from the routines and worries of daily life. Engaging in passion pursuits purely for the joy of them provides a sense of escapism and tranquility, which in turn can lead to reduced stress levels and improving our overall mood.

Whether it's the calm concentration required for painting, the physical exertion of a dance class, or the intellectual challenge of writing a book, each hobby offers a unique way to decompress and find a calming balance.

Adding a new hobby or interest has not only enriched my personal life, it has also had a ripple effect on those around me. Sharing my inspiration with friends, family, and acquaintances has encouraged others to explore their own interests.

NEWS AND CURRENT AFFAIRS

Maintaining an awareness of current events and global happenings via news sites and podcasts has added a surprising depth to my life as I've grown older. It's not merely about the advantage of being informed; staying on top of the news has also given me many meaningful interactions with people far beyond my ordinary social network.

Whether shopping, commuting, or engaging in everyday activities, my grasp of current news has even been a conduit for connecting with people I serendipitously meet and strike up a conversation with.

These mostly spontaneous exchanges allow for hearing and bridging differing viewpoints, cultivating mutual understanding and respectful conversations. Exploring discussions about the latest news doesn't just expand my worldview; it strengthens my sense of awareness and belonging.

My awareness of current events and global happenings provides me with a mental workout, similar to the benefits I get from physical exercise. My ability to grasp complex world events feels sharper.

SETTING GOALS

Setting goals has become a cornerstone of my approach to aging and staying engaged with the world around me. It's not just about listing desires or achievements I hope to tick off my bucket list; it's a profound exercise in introspection and forward planning.

By thoughtfully considering what I want to achieve in the near and distant future, I not only give myself a roadmap to follow but also instill a sense of purpose that fuels my daily life. Whether it's keeping me physically healthy, maintaining relationships, or working towards completing a creative project, each goal is a guiding light that helps me navigate what's important in life.

Regular goal setting encourages me to reflect on my values and how they translate into tangible objectives. This alignment between values and goals ensures that my pursuits are meaningful and resonate with my deeper self. It's not just about achieving for the sake of achievement; it's about growth, learning, and exploration.

For instance, setting a goal to learn a new language or volunteering for a cause I care about enriches my life in ways that mere material success cannot. It connects me to new ideas, and people, expanding my worldview and enhancing my empathy and understanding.

The process of setting and working towards goals keeps me mentally and emotionally agile. Each challenge, regardless really if

I succeed or fail, offers invaluable lessons and builds resilience and helps me maintain a decent level of adaptability. I firmly believe this to be particularly valuable at this stage of my life, where change becomes one of the few constants.

The goals I set act as milestones, motivating me to push further. They imbue my life with a narrative arc, transforming the aging process from a series of losses into a often fascinating experience filled with both growth and discovery.

I think it's important to approach goal setting with flexibility and kindness towards oneself. Not all goals will be met, and that's okay. Life's unpredictability means that adaptability is as much a virtue as it is determination.

Some goals may evolve or even be replaced by more relevant aspirations as my circumstances shift. Adaptability is certainly a strength and it allows me to remain relevant and engaged in the world around me. As I see it, it's not the attainment of goals that ultimately defines our lives, but the journey we undertake to pursue them. This journey, fueled by aspirations and moderated by our experience, keeps us moving forward, eager to see what each new day brings.

In essence, setting goals is more than a simple strategy – it's a blueprint for a more fulfilling life. It's about creating a life that reflects our deepest desires and values, a life that challenges us to grow and adapt, and a life that is rich with experiences and connections.

As I look ahead, I see not just the goals I aim to achieve but the person I hope to become: someone who lives fully, loves deeply, and leaves a positive mark on the world.

Staying relevant as we age requires a proactive approach to personal growth, maintaining connections, and adapting to change. Ultimately, relevance is determined not only by your age but by your willingness to stay engaged with people (and possibly a pet) and make an effort to be a positive force in the world around you.

The Aging Man's Survival Guide

DEALING WITH DENIAL & MORTALITY

Thoughts and strategies for enjoying
more of the path forward.

As the book's final chapter, my ambition with this epilogue is to emphasize the importance of acknowledging the aging process and eventually accepting our mortality – not merely just to come to terms with dying or with death itself, but as a means to remind us to embrace the time we have left and, ultimately, make the most of it.

Accepting that my time is limited has helped me refocus my energy to nurture healthier relationships (and to discard detrimental ones), to setting new personal goals, and living life with wholehearted passion.

Through personal anecdotes and heartfelt thoughts, my ambition with the following pages is to inspire you to recognize the beauty and urgency of each day and to encourage you to lead a life brimming with purpose and a wealth of enjoyable social interactions.

Included are practical methods and strategies for how to accept the inevitability of life's closing phase and the importance of organizing and communicating end-of-life wishes. I'll also discuss why assigning a Power of Attorney and an Executor is important, alongside with managing your digital legacy.

Life Reflections

Now and again, increasingly so, I take time to reflect on my journey, my accomplishments, and the abounding buffet of life experiences I've racked up in my 60 plus years on this wondrous planet.

I'm a firm believer that by focusing on the more positive moments – yet also acknowledging some of the challenges that I've overcome and survived, I feel a roughly equal amount of amazement and satisfaction about how well my life has turned out so far.

Fortunately, my mind has a great ability to recall many of life's highlights. Though not entirely erased, the majority of my most traumatic experiences, primarily related to the unforeseen deaths of loved ones, accidents that impacted my life's trajectory as well as scarring childhood memories, are fortunately fuzzy and faded.

PARENTING

Parenthood has by far been my life's most adventurous experience. I initially approached the idea of becoming a father with a lot of skepticism, shaped in no small way by the wounds from a childhood marred by my mother's alcoholism and my father's abandonment. These early experiences left me questioning my capability to provide a stable, nurturing environment for a child.

But despite my initial doubts and lack of confidence, the moment I became a father, the very first time I saw my newborn daughter, a profound transformation ensued. The first few years were certainly a strange mix of joy and worry, but for every birthday my daughter celebrated, I secretly rejoiced in victory over my fears of repeating my parents' abysmal mistakes.

As my daughter grew, so did the complexities of parenting, pushing me to learn and adapt. I had never had any role models, so at least on a practical level, I was often improvising. Through this now 24 year journey, which has mostly been smooth thanks to my wife Charlotte, a stable, emotionally grounded Swedish woman, I've discovered strengths I really didn't think I had – as well as patience, and above all, a surprising ability to provide an almost infinite amount of unconditional love to our daughter.

My skepticism has been transformed into a testament of the transformative power of love and of breaking free from the shadows of my childhood and the constraints it had on me for so long.

So, parenthood is easily my greatest accomplishment. Today, our adult daughter Elle Agnes is a beautiful, independent young woman who shapes her own life, overcoming challenges with strength, confidence, and persistence rooted in the love we've done our best to provide.

ASPIRATIONS AND DISTRACTIONS

Since turning 60, I've holstered some of my more outlandish ambitions and outlined a few reasonably achievable goals that feel right for this stage of life. Even if my career as a freelance creative is coming to a close, having new, meaningful plans and projects seems to provide me with a positive sense of purpose and motivation. If you've started reading this book here, there's more of this topic in the chapters **Designing Retirement, Staying Relevant** and, **Brighter Days Ahead.**

Bluntly put, by creating a "bucket list" with new things you want to learn, places you want to visit and experiences you hope to add to your life – before too long – can be just the distraction you need from the at times daunting reminders of aging.

I try to keep in mind that a bucket list does not necessarily have to be elaborate or filled with extraordinarily adventurous trips or high-flown ambitions. Since simple goals are usually more reachable – yet can be just as rewarding – my list is a mix of both achievable dreams and realistic aspirations.

It's important that we don't hesitate to try new things, including new hobbies and interests which for whatever reason may have been put off earlier in life, even when it looks like the learning curve has become increasingly steep.

At this age in life, I know it's essential for me not to shy away from changes and challenges that have the potential to make a profoundly positive impact on my life.

LEARNING NEW STUFF

Though cognitive functions and motor skills naturally slow down as we age, our brain's capacity for neuroplasticity – its ability to form new neural connections – remains intact. By leveraging accumulated physical and mental experiences, we can continue to learn new stuff regardless of how old we are.

Whether it's learning how to navigate a new city, a new language or trying out a new sport, engaging in physical and mental activities will encourage the growth of new neural pathways. So, as long as we keep challenging ourselves, we can enjoy both cognitive growth and physical vitality for the rest of our lives.

Physically Active = Mentally Healthy

For me, there are no vitamins or elixirs more effective than integrating some form of physical exercise into my daily life. By regularly going to the gym, jogging or just taking a long walk vastly improves my mental and emotional well-being.

The reverse is also true. I tend to get stuck in a mental quagmire if I don't engage in some kind of physical activity – preferably where I break a sweat at least a few times a week.

While it might not necessarily help clear all the clouds or suppress periodic thoughts about my mortality or keep all chronic, age-related ailments away, I know that exercise will definitely increase the overall quality of my life as I age.

STAY CONNECTED

There is reliable research suggesting that as we grow older, maintaining a socially active life with old friends as well as gaining new acquaintances, can promote good mental and emotional health.

Being active as a physically present participant in a community or group of fellow hobbyists and maintaining contact with friends and neighbors can provide a health-inducing sense of belonging and by extension, an appreciation of life.

While being part of online social groups certainly offers global reach in realtime with likeminded individuals from the comfort of home, I've also experienced how this kind of social interactivity can lead to contention, conflicts and stress. Not to mention risk of an unhealthy social media fixation, which I've mentioned in the chapter **Staying Relevant.**

Here, dear reader, I must reiterate from the chapter **Improving & Extending Life**, as you likely already know, stress triggers the production of the hormone cortisol. And while cortisol is crucial for managing short-term stress effectively, chronic or prolonged stress can lead to persistently elevated cortisol levels. This can have some very negative effects on our health and be especially detrimental as we age.

Chronic stress can actually contribute to conditions like anxiety, depression, sleep disturbances, weight gain, and impaired immune function.

MY EMOTIONAL LEGACY

From time to time, I find myself reflecting on the legacy I wish to leave behind in the minds and hearts of family, relatives, and friends. In these subtle and humble moments of soul-searching and contemplation, whether it's as a reliable friend, a supportive partner, or simply a reasonably good parent, I hope to be remembered as someone who participated and added something in a meaningful way to their lives.

As I age, I hope to be able to continue to be close to those that matter most to me and maybe even deepen our relationships. Likewise, as brutal as it may sound, I have realized how important it is for me to not waste my time and my love on people, regardless of how we are connected, that don't somehow actively contribute to my life emotionally or who see our relationship as more peripheral than essential.

I want to be remembered for the shared laughter, the inspiration, the silences, and the supportive talks in times of need. The warmth others feel when they think of me, and possibly a feeling of love when my name is spoken. That would be a nice emotional legacy to leave behind.

SPIRITUALITY AND PHILOSOPHY

Many seek comfort in aging by studying spiritual beliefs or engaging in philosophical contemplation in order to better understand and possibly find answers to the profound questions that relate to life, death and thoughts about a possible afterlife.

This introspective journey can be both healthy and somewhat unsettling. Sure, this path can serve as a source of comfort, providing a framework through which we can make sense of the complexities of our existence.

BUT IT MIGHT ALSO ADD INSECURITY AND WORRY AND STRESS.

After all, what happens happens and there is so far not much conclusive evidence to suggest that whatever what we believe in will actually have any impact on what happens once our final breath has left our body.

Regardless of what, how or on to whom we lean, researching different perspectives can still provide a most interesting personal voyage. A voyage that offers not only solace but perhaps also a profound link to some of the theories aiming to explain the mysteries of life and death.

ACCEPTANCE

In my experience, we men, especially as we get older, typically shy away from discussing heavy topics like health, dying and death. This reservedness can obviously prevent us from coming to terms with our own mortality.

If thinking about the end of life and the existential implications that come with these thoughts create anxiety or even depression, it's probably time to consider getting some professional help.

Support can be sought from several different sources: including a psychologist, a psychiatrist, theological experts (including nuns and priests) specializing in end-of-life therapy as well as open conversations with close friends and family members.

Professionals within the field of existentialism have the expertise to help us navigate the complex emotions and questions that arise by offering a dialogue that can lead to a deeper understanding, clarity, acceptance and hopefully peace of mind. A skilled therapist, combined with the support from conversations with friends and family, can be invaluable.

By sharing our fears and feelings we can demystify or at least downplay the topic of death, which can help us build a stronger understanding and acceptance of life's inevitable end.

MY PATH FORWARD

Regardless of religious belief, whether we subscribe to atheism or take an agnostic approach to the eventual existence of celestial beings and the much-hyped but unsubstantiated afterlife, at some point, we'll have to concede that all living things have an expiration date.

My personal mantra has long been: I believe in life before death.

Taboo as it is to some, I do not believe that dedicating a thought now and then about death or dying is negative or distressing. Nor do I think it's counter productive or that by thinking about it will somehow jinx me. Superstition is religion's closest neighbor, and I tend to keep a fair distance from both.

Fact is, at this stage of my life, I find that by allowing thoughts of mortality to flow freely through and within me – but without dwelling so much that I feel distraught or get melancholic – once they've left, I feel I can achieve an even stronger focus on what I want to accomplish and experience before the shifty Grim Reaper does come a knockin'.

That said, in situations where there seems to be a certain level of risk that death could at least theoretically be near, I'd be lying if I didn't admit that unsound thoughts about mortality have bounced around in my mind.

But even when I've sat in an old bush plane during a thunderstorm, or, been jostled about in the backseat of a rickety taxi while speeding down a busy highway (in torrential rain), within that temporary anxiety lies a sense of consolation in knowing that things can only get so bad.

That though cut shorter than I had expected, just like every other organic thing on our planet, I have arrived at a place and a moment where I have to check out, take a curtain call and, time allowing, bid adieu.

Hopefully, I'll be able to remember that up to that very point, my life had been a mostly fascinating experience.

On the other hand, should I make it to eighty or even ninety and beyond, I suppose that leaving the party won't be such a bad thing. At least not if I realize I'm no longer participating very well. Or worse yet, if the other guests at the party feel that I have long overstayed my welcome.

Some of my friends with elderly parents have implied that they are tired of caring for them and might just secretly yearn for when they no longer have to. Though I've never heard anyone be so verbally blunt or outspoken about this most sensitive topic, I have seen unmistakable allusions, telling facial expression and abysmally deep sighs.

My own parents died when I was quite young and as tragic as that definitely was, the only silver lining is that I don't have to deal with their geriatric phase of life. I can only hope that my daughter or wife won't have to be too burdened once I become unable to take care of myself.

As morbid as this may sound, eventually, one of the silver linings of getting older could actually be death itself.

I mean, that at some stage, possibly as soon as once you've turned 60, you begin to discover in the deep depths of your inner mind that there is a kernel of solace in knowing that you will eventually not have to deal with some of life's unavoidable crap.

This especially if you are no longer able to enjoy most of the fun stuff that makes life so worth living. Like eating great food, having sex, and traveling.

Maybe later on, if and when we become fully cognizant that our number's comings up, hopefully sooner than later, we might even embrace the thought of checking out.

A part of getting older has been to at least try to come to terms with my own mortality and accumulating both courage and solace.

Here are some strategies that have helped me along the way.

ACKNOWLEDGE AND ACCEPT

No matter how much you worry about it and regardless of how healthy you've lived your life, how much wealth you've amassed, death is still going to happen. Death is the only real democratizer. While it takes no hostages, the inescapability of mortality has come to actually offer me some solace since there's really no point at all in getting too worked up about it. Like me, I assume most hope that when it does occur, it will at least not be too outdrawn and or painful, or messy.

DON'T STRESS. IT'S GOING TO BE A MESS ANYWAY.

Not that it really matters since we'll be dead anyway. But the fact is that following our last breath and heartbeat, all our body's muscles will contract relax, relieving all tension in our cadaver, including our bowel and bladder.

This less-than-pleasant revelation has me contemplating the proactive step of donning adult diapers as soon as I feel or am told that the end is near. It's about leaving behind a clean scene for whoever finds me. I like to consider it a thoughtful, albeit unconventional, last gesture of kindness!

CAUSE OF DEATH

For the past few years, whenever I hear about someone close to my age dying, I became almost obsessively curious with how and why the person died. Aside from terminal illness, suicide and really bad luck, for me, the worst possible scenario is if the person in question was healthy and fit and how some vital part of the individual's body, for whatever reason, just gave up. Poof!

In those rare cases, I tend to dwell on my own mortality and simulate way beyond a reasonable amount of time, that I, a relatively fit and healthy sixty year-old, could also abruptly die just as suddenly as the deceased I was reading about.

Conversely, I am utterly relieved, albeit with a brew of guilt and glee, whenever I learn that there was some medical explanation or underlying condition, perhaps a disease or poor lifestyle habits, as a direct or indirect cause of death.

While working out at my local gym some time ago, a guy my age fell off the treadmill he was running on and collapsed. He was pronounced DOA once the ambulance had parked outside the ICU at the nearest hospital. I never found out what caused his sudden death and whenever I think about it, particularly when I'm on one of the gym's treadmills, possibly even the very machine the poor fellow was exercising on, not knowing continues to bother me.

While navigating thoughts about life and death is something I am certain most people do at some point in their lives, sharing these feelings with family, and loved ones can provide emotional support and above all, increase our understanding that we are not alone in tackling mortality.

MACHISMO

For a slew of reasons, most of which I believe have been addressed in the chapter **Health Secrecy**, we men tend not to talk much about the unpredictability of what is arguably life's most profoundly unsolvable mystery, how, when and where we die.

Through film, literature and music, a man's death is mostly described and dramatized as a phase filled with machismo calm acceptance, bravery, heroism, or, at the very least, some level of stoicism.

In reality, when we die, for many of us, it's going to be a shocking, painful, lonesome affair. Which makes it all the more important to talk openly about it beforehand in order to feel some kind of comfort from the collective.

I've found consolation about my own mortality by talking with people considerably older than I am and when appropriate, getting their take on how to deal with their own death.

EUTHANASIA

In a scenario where you are terminally ill beyond medical treatment and where maybe you are no longer coherent or even conscious, assisted dying can be an option. However, keep in mind that this introduces complex legal considerations. Laws pertaining to euthanasia vary significantly by country and jurisdiction.

In some countries including Belgium, the Netherlands, and Canada, euthanasia or physician-assisted suicide is currently legal under specific conditions, allowing individuals facing incurable illnesses and significant suffering to choose a dignified death under close medical supervision. These laws typically require rigorous consent procedures, that can comprise of psychiatric evaluations and multiple confirmations of a patient's wishes.

In many parts of the world, euthanasia is illegal and in some countries there's an ongoing ethical, moral, and religious debate about the right to choose how and when to die. For people living in countries where euthanasia is not an option, detailing wishes about the withdrawal or withholding of life-sustaining treatment becomes even more important.

Understanding the legal landscape of euthanasia and assisted dying in your country and incorporating preferences into your Advance Directives can make sure that end-of-life care respects your wishes, within the bounds of the law in which you live under.

Countries where euthanasia is currently legal and where foreigners can take advantage of current laws about physician-assisted suicide:

CANADA: Broad legal framework for medically assisted dying for individuals meeting certain conditions, including serious and incurable illness, disease, or disability.

BELGIUM: Euthanasia is legal for individuals experiencing unbearable physical or mental suffering with no prospect of improvement. Foreigners have been granted access to euthanasia, provided they meet the stringent legal requirements.

THE NETHERLANDS: Legalized both euthanasia and physician-assisted suicide under strict conditions, including unbearable suffering with no prospect of improvement. There have been cases where non-residents with terminal illnesses have sought and undergone euthanasia, though this is rare and involves a complex legal process.

LUXEMBOURG: Allows euthanasia and assisted suicide for adults who are in a condition of advanced incurable illness or unbearable suffering.

SWITZERLAND: Assisted suicide is legal, provided the individual assists themselves and the helper has no selfish motives. Organizations like Dignitas offer assisted suicide to non-residents who meet their criteria

SPAIN: Legalized euthanasia and assisted suicide for individuals with serious and incurable diseases causing unbearable suffering.

COLOMBIA: Euthanasia is legal for terminally ill patients experiencing intense suffering.

NEW ZEALAND: The End of Life Choice Act allows assisted dying for terminally ill people with less than 6 months to live.

PORTUGAL: Parliament passed laws to legalize euthanasia and assisted suicide, but specifics of implementation may vary.

GERMANY: The Constitutional Court ruled that the right to a self-determined death includes the freedom to seek assistance from third parties, leading to partial decriminalization of assisted suicide.

AUSTRALIA: Assisted dying laws vary by state, with Victoria, Western Australia, Tasmania, South Australia, and Queensland having legislation allowing it under specific conditions. Plan for End-of-Life Matters

The prospect of addressing practical things related to my own death, like drafting a will, detailing end-of-life wishes, and planning my funeral are inherently a strange and even distressing activity. Still, undertaking them in advance has proven to provide me with a profound sense of control – and by extension, given me some peace of mind.

By proactively engaging rationally with these aspects of life, I am not only sure that my wishes are clearly laid out and documented, I find comfort in knowing that I will also leave behind a somewhat structured and thoughtful roadmap for my loved ones to follow.

Embracing practical considerations reflects a responsible approach to the inevitable. And acknowledging the importance of preparedness – while still offering some comfort for both myself and those who will fulfill my decisions in the future – might add to a more heartfelt remembrance of me.

Writing a will, detailing a testament, and specifying final wishes for funeral arrangements, can give you and your loved ones peace of mind. While it might seem morbid or depressing to think about it right now, there are several reasons why it's important to plan ahead, especially once you've reached the age of 60.

HERE ARE SOME THINGS TO CONSIDER

WILL AND TESTAMENT

I could argue against the necessity of drafting a will and testament from the perspective that emphasizes the ultimate irrelevance of my worldly possessions after I've died.

From this viewpoint, the process of listing and dividing my assets seems futile using the, "I couldn't take them with me, so why should I give a damn who gets them once I'm gone?" argument. For some, it might even be tempting to imagine leaving a legacy of chaos as a final statement, or, as a means of twisted revenge.

The reality is that the fallout affects those left behind much more than we might be able to understand and appreciate. It makes sense that the emotional toll of unresolved estate issues can exacerbate the grief of loss, leaving loved ones to deal with a lot of practical problems to solve, most of which could have been avoided with some foresight and planning.

On the other hand, some might see the absence of a will as a statement of detachment from material possessions, suggesting a philosophical stance that value is not placed in physical wealth but rather in the intangibles left behind.

However, my main argument for having a will and testament is rooted in a desire to prevent potential disputes and ensure that my wishes are respected after I die. Without a clear will, the process of distributing my assets can become a source of significant conflict among surviving family members, leading to strained relationships and, in some extreme cases, lengthy legal battles.

It's important to keep in mind that a will and testament can protect the interests of minor children, dependents with special needs, or even friends and charities that might otherwise be overlooked in a standard legal distribution process.

A will serves as my voice from beyond, guiding the allocation of assets in a way that reflects my intentions. It can also serve as a final act of care and consideration, reducing the administrative and legal process surrounding asset distribution, potentially saving time, money, and heartache for everyone involved.

ASSET DISTRIBUTION

Firstly, consider the unique needs of your family when planning the distribution of your assets. This might involve making specific provisions for minors, individuals with special needs, or family members who have been particularly supportive.

You might also want to consider the impact of your financial support on their lives, ensuring it brings benefit rather than unintended financial stress. For instance, setting up a trust fund can provide a controlled flow of money to beneficiaries who may not be ready or able to manage a lump sum effectively.

For items of sentimental value or family heirlooms, specifying who should receive these can prevent disagreements and souring relationships. Think not so much of the monetary value as much as of the emotional significance these items might provide.

By communicating your wishes, either through your will or a

personal letter, you can ensure that these assets go to those who will value them most.

In situations where you wish to support charitable causes, specifying donations in your will can be a powerful way to extend your legacy beyond your family. This can serve as a valuable example of generosity and civic responsibility for your heirs.

Finally, it's wise to engage in open conversations with your family about your estate planning. While discussing death and inheritance can be sensitive and uncomfortable, transparent communication can minimize misunderstandings and help prepare your family for their roles and responsibilities.

It also offers an opportunity to explain the reasoning behind your decisions, which can be especially important in cases where the distribution may not seem equal but is equitable based on individual needs and circumstances.

GUARDIANSHIP

Guardianship involves legally designating an individual or individuals whom you trust to take over the responsibility of caring for your dependents, making decisions about their education, healthcare, and daily living needs.

Appointing a guardian for your dependents is a profound expression of love and care and makes sure that they continue to thrive under the guardianship of someone who shares your values and concerns for their wellbeing.

The process of selecting a guardian should be done with great care, considering the potential guardian's values, parenting style, financial stability, and the emotional bond they have with your dependents. It's also important to have open and honest discussions with those you are considering as guardians to ensure they are willing and able to take on this significant responsibility.

In addition to naming a primary guardian, it's wise to appoint a secondary guardian as a contingency in case the primary guardian is unable to fulfill their duties. This provides an extra layer of protection for your dependents.

Legal documentation is essential in the guardianship appointment process. By working with a legal professional, you'll be guided through the necessary steps to make sure your wishes are documented and legally binding. This not only provides you with peace of mind but also helps prevent potential legal disputes among family members or other interested parties.

FUNERAL AND BURIAL WISHES

BURIAL VS. CREMATION

To make sure your wishes are respected, I strongly suggest that you clearly state your preference for cremation or burial beforehand. it's typically not recommended to solely rely on including them in a will, as it might be read too late.

Instead, consider pre-need planning with a funeral home, creating a separate document, a letter of instruction or communicating directly with loved ones. Consulting with an estate planner can also help you choose the best approach for documenting your wishes.

If burial, consider specifying the cemetery or type of burial plot you prefer. If cremation, indicate what you want to be done with the ashes. It's become increasingly popular to spread ashes of loved ones in unconventional locations, including during rides at Disneyland, from the rooftops of famous skyscrapers and in public parks.

Consider that if your choice of where you wish your ashes to be strewn is not allowed or even against the law, the potential legal consequences might hinder your instructions from being carried out.

SPECIFIC REQUESTS

Including special requests for your funeral service can transform it from a traditional ceremony into a memorable, deeply personal reflection of the life you've lived. Specific texts, whether they are favorite passages from literature, lines from cherished songs, or excerpts from religious texts, can resonate deeply with those you've invited, evoking memories and emotions that capture who they remember you as.

Music, too, can play a pivotal role in personalizing your funeral service. Songs that you enjoyed, a classic pop song, a rock anthem or maybe a jazz standard, can serve as a powerful tribute, encapsulating the soundtrack of your life.

Beyond texts and music, other personal touches can include the display of photographs, personal items, or a short film that chronicles a part of your life. You can even choose to have a theme that reflects a passion, like an exhibit of your passions.

Think of it this way; adding personal items and specific requests can serve as a soothing celebration of who you were, your interests, your achievements, and the love you shared with those around you. By easing the grieving process you will also make sure that your legacy is remembered and cherished in a way that is true to your spirit.

FUNERAL COSTS

Since funeral expenses can reach substantial amounts, depending on how specific you have been with requests of burial, venue, number of guests, food etc, setting aside enough funds can be a practical and thoughtful way to ease the potential stress on your loved ones during a time of grief.

By investing in a prepaid funeral plan, you can be sure that the costs associated with your final farewell are taken care of in advance. This foresight not only spares your family from the financial strain, it also allows them to focus on mourning and celebrating your life without the added pressure of managing expenses.

Whether it's through a savings account designated for this purpose, a life insurance policy, or a funeral insurance plan, preparing for inevitable costs is a compassionate way to show care for your family's well-being.

LEGAL AND MEDICAL DIRECTIVES

CREATING AN ADVANCE DIRECTIVE & LIVING WILL

Articulating your wishes for medical treatment in scenarios where you are unable to make decisions for yourself is an important part of end-of-life planning. You can create this through so-called Advance Directives or a Living Will, documents that specify your preferences for medical interventions, including the use of medication, life support systems, and other life-sustaining measures.

By clearly stating your wishes in these legally binding documents, you offer a guide for your family and healthcare providers, which can be particularly comforting in stressful situations where difficult decisions have to be made.

POWER OF ATTORNEY

Basically, this is about appointing someone to make legal and financial decisions on your behalf if you become incapacitated. The concept of a Power of Attorney (POA) can play an important role in planning for life's unforeseen twists and turns.

By appointing a trusted individual to make legal and financial decisions on your behalf, a POA makes sure that your affairs are managed according to your wishes, even if you become unable to do so yourself.

This is a legal "instrument" that allows you to choose someone who understands your preferences and acts in your best interests, providing peace of mind to both you and your loved ones.

Whether it's managing your investments, paying your bills, or making critical medical decisions, a POA should be an essential part of your retirement plan. Beyond its practical benefits, establishing a POA is also a gesture of trust and foresight, reflecting a thoughtful consideration for your future and the well-being of those you care about.

Without a POA, your loved ones might have to go through court proceedings to obtain the authority to manage your affairs, a situation that can be avoided with this proactive step.

APPOINTING AN EXECUTOR

An Executor is a key person appointed through a will to manage and settle the estate of someone that has died. The Executor primary role is to ensure the decedent's final wishes are fulfilled and these duties can range from gathering the estate's assets, paying off debts and taxes, to distributing what remains to the beneficiaries as outlined in the will.

This role demands trustworthiness, organizational skills, and a good grasp of legal and financial matters due to the involvement in the process and potential disputes among inheritors.

The presence of an executor is vital for the clear legal management of the estate, timely payment of obligations, and the proper execution of the will's directives. Choosing a reliable and competent executor, along with an alternate, is an important aspect of estate planning, as it guarantees that one's legacy is preserved and distributed in accordance with their wishes.

DIGITAL LEGACY

In the digital age we live in today, our online presence and digital assets have become an integral part of who we are, which warrants some considerations. Digital legacy planning involves specifying instructions for how you want your digital assets –ranging from social media accounts and email to digital files, photographs, and even cryptocurrencies – to be handled after your passing.

This not only ensures that your digital footprint is managed according to your wishes but also simplifies the process for your loved ones to access, memorialize, or close your online accounts.

Communicating these directives through your will, provides a clear roadmap for the Executor of your estate, preventing potential disputes and protecting your online identity. By taking control of your digital legacy preemptively, you ensure that your memories and assets stored in the digital realm are preserved or disposed of appropriately, echoing your values and preferences.

As you close this chapter, I hope my thoughts on aging and mortality and life's richness have resonated with you. Accepting death as an inevitable part of life is not just about preparing for the end but also about embracing and enhancing the quality of our lives right now.

This book is an invitation to view the inevitability of death not with denial or fear, but as a motivating force to live more fully and leave a meaningful legacy. May we all find comfort in knowing that in accepting our mortality, we are actually embracing life here and now.

OTHER BOOKS BY
JOAKIM LLOYD RABOFF

Västra Hamnen 2005	2005	9789163172632
Svenskar i thailand	2006	9789163185496
Västra Hamnen 2007	2007	9789163197345
Västra Hamnen 2008	2008	9789197750103
Västra Hamnen 2009	2009	9789197810333
Västra Hamnen 2010	2010	9789163364891
Västra Hamnen 2011	2011	9789163384813
Västra Hamnen 2012	2012	9789197810302
Västra Hamnen 2013	2013	9789197810319
Västra Hamnen 2014	2014	9789198179507
Vad sysslar du med?	2014	9789163361555
Västra Hamnen 2015	2015	9789198249408
Turning torso I	2015	9789163790089
Turning Torso II	2017	9789151918617
Vi är Malmö Opera	2017	9789163934360
Ögonblick från Vejbystrand	2020	9789151948867
Sliperiet i Gylsboda	2021	9789152705896
New York City	2023	9789198852134
Heavy Metal Talat Noi's Sieng Gong	2003	9789198852103
Silhouette Surfers	2023	9789198852110
Resurfaced	2003	9789198852127
Västra Hamnen 2004-2024	2024	9789198852141

Milton Keynes UK
Ingram Content Group UK Ltd.
UKHW020640010824
446326UK00013B/402